Running from Perfection

Praise for *Running from Perfection*

"Blending personal narrative with scientific insight, this book is a powerful testament to the resilience of the human spirit. For anyone who has struggled with perfectionism, self-doubt, or the search for meaning, this is a story of hope, perseverance, and the transformative power of movement in the great outdoors."

—Hillary Allen, professional ultrarunner and author of *Out and Back: A Runner's Story of Survival Against All Odds*

"Caitlin's powerful story is a must-read for anyone touched by eating disorders or mental health issues. Her experience highlights the profound impact of nature and physical activity on recovery."

—Chad Lasater, Master's American record holder and UESCA-certified ultrarunning coach

"A gripping blend of memoir and neuroscience—insightful, inspiring, and deeply human."

—Sarah Williams, adventurer and host of the *Tough Girl Podcast*

"In *Running from Perfection*, Caitlin offers a unique insight into the world of disordered eating as she intertwines her personal story with her neuroscience practice. Caitlin's resilience is inspiring, and this book empowers the reader to allow themself more grace in daily life!"

—Bridget Storm, corporate clinical dietitian

"In *Running from Perfection*, Dr. Massone helps those struggling with eating disorders understand their faulty wiring. With a neuroscientist's expertise and a patient's experience, she takes the reader on her journey from self-loathing to self-love by connecting to the natural world. An important addition to our understanding of eating disorders."

—Shannon Payne, PhD, ultrarunner and geneticist

RUNNING FROM PERFECTION

My Journey from Eating Disorders to Endurance Sports— and the Neuroscience Behind It

Caitlin Massone, MD

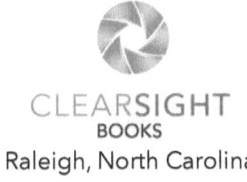

CLEARSIGHT BOOKS
Raleigh, North Carolina

Copyright 2025 Caitlin Massone
All rights reserved. Copying or use of this material without express written consent by author is prohibited by law.

ISBN paperback: 978-1-945209-54-3
ISBN ebook: 978-1-945209-55-0
Library of Congress Control Number: 2025903877

Published by Clear Sight Books, Raleigh, North Carolina
Cover design by Howard Grossman

For my mom, Kerin, and Stephen

Contents

A Note to the Reader xi
Introduction 1
Chapter 1. Little Miss Perfect 7
Chapter 2. Perfect Storm 21
Chapter 3. Nature + Nurture + Stress 35
Chapter 4. The Icing on the Cake 49
Chapter 5. Vanishing Act 61
Chapter 6. The Chemistry of Contentment 71
Chapter 7. Making the Cut 85
Chapter 8. The Invisible Monster 95
Chapter 9. Practice Makes Perfect 107
Chapter 10. The Mountains Are Calling 117
Chapter 11. Recovery Is a Marathon, Not a Sprint 127
Chapter 12. Perfect Match 141
Chapter 13. Running from Perfection 151
Chapter 14. Type II Fun 161
Chapter 15. Exercise Junkie 173
Chapter 16. A New High 185
Chapter 17. Above the Clouds 195
Chapter 18. Into the Forest I Go 209
Chapter 19. The Perfect Test 221
Chapter 20. Fifty Miles 231
Afterword 239
Acknowledgments 245
Notes 247
Resources 251

A Note to the Reader

My goal in writing this book is to provide some insight into the mind of a person who has lived through a chronic eating disorder, including personal thoughts and reflections as well as scientific discussion of the brain changes that occur. I discuss topics such as addiction, the formation of habits in the brain, the genetics and neurobiology of eating disorders, and the effects of running and nature on mental health.

When referring to statistics on eating disorders in athletes, the binary "male" and "female" are used. This is not intended to be exclusionary but is rather based on the data reported in recent studies comparing these groups. Although I felt defined by my illness and often referred to myself as "anorexic" or "bulimic," I have attempted to use language such as "person with anorexia" or "people experiencing bulimia" in an effort to emphasize that an eating disorder is indeed a disease and need not be one's sole or permanent identity.

While I am a board-certified neurologist, well versed in neuroanatomy and neurochemistry, I am not a psychiatrist or psychologist. I am not an expert on eating disorders and their treatment. This writing reflects my personal experience and unconventional recovery from eating disorders through participating in endurance sports and rediscovering the healing power of nature.

My experience is not generalizable to every person with an eating disorder, and my opinions are not a recommendation on how to recover from an eating disorder. Each person has an individualized path, and many people living with eating disorders need the help of therapists, counselors, physicians, coaches, parents, and nutritionists on their road to recovery. Some may also benefit from the use of psychiatric medications and other adjunctive therapies.

Parents, teachers, coaches, and athletes, I hope my story raises awareness of the signs and symptoms of an eating disorder in a young person and empowers you to help that person in need.

INTRODUCTION

I'm standing on the summit of Mount Rainier. It's 5:10 a.m., earlier than I wake up for work, but the last hour of feverish climbing to the top was more invigorating than a double espresso, and I feel wide awake. Three time zones to the east, my husband and mother are anxiously awaiting a text to know that I've made it. There hasn't been cell service for hours, and I feel so far removed from civilization, so focused on the climb, that it's odd to even try to use my phone. My fingers move ineptly across the screen. "Holy shit! I'm at the summit!" I send to both, hoping at least one will receive my message. The blue progress bar at the top of my iPhone is as frozen as my fingers, already chilled from the brief exposure to the cold air. I tuck my hands back into heavy winter gloves.

The summit team gathers in the darkness of the crater, protected from the 10°F windchill and the gusts that whip around the top of the volcano. It is surprisingly still in the crater, and warm, a reminder of what lies deep beneath the snow-crusted surface we're sitting on. Just around the lip of the crater is an expansive view of the Cascade Range and the start of a magnificent sunrise. Glowing streams of red and orange melt across the horizon, like paint being poured across a black canvas. Soon the morning sun will highlight the path back down the mountain, and I'll be able to see all the frightening drop-offs and crevasses we passed on the moonlit ascent. I feel breathless, struck by the beauty of the landscape and the effects of the altitude and an effortful climb. My gloved hands clumsily pull my puffy parka tight around my core, and I nestle into its warmth.

This is the crux of a three-day mountaineering trip—two days of trekking in mountaineering boots and crampons, and one long overnight push to get to the top of this iconic glaciated mountain. Most people have heard of Mount Rainier, even if they have never seen it or climbed it. For an aspiring mountaineer, it is a coveted peak that opens doors to bigger mountains, higher altitudes, and dreams of climbing Denali or Mount Everest.

Six hours of constant movement and exertion in the dark and we've finally made it. I have never felt so powerful and proud of my body as I do in this moment. I was able to push through the discomfort and fatigue that accumulated in my muscles over three days and countless steps forward. And my mind was able to convince my muscles to keep working when they wanted to quit. Blistered feet, sore shoulders from the gravitational force of a 50-pound backpack, burning calves from the relentless stair-climber of snow, rock, and volcanic scree. The mental resilience I've worked for has paid off.

In the months leading up to the climb, I ran long distance after long distance and scrambled up and down the walls of the climbing gym. In the years before that, I slowly molded myself into an endurance athlete: first a runner and then a mountaineer. My running journey started with a few miles; a few miles turned into a half-marathon, then a marathon, then an ultramarathon. A never-ending game of testing limits, seeing

INTRODUCTION

how much further I could push through physical pain using mental fortitude and determination. Solid, muscular calves and quads are proof of how many miles I've accumulated along the way. But I had to start from scratch, to learn to love my body again after I nearly destroyed it, and my confidence as a runner lagged behind a growing pile of finisher's medals.

I always had the potential to be an athlete, from the first time I kicked a soccer ball at the age of five, but for too many years, I lost sight of that. I shamed my body for being strong. I leveled it with a wrecking ball. It took decades to fully rebuild it, to undo the damage I did, to break the destructive habits that broke me. In reality, it isn't a three-day climb that has brought me to the top of Mount Rainier but rather a twenty-year journey.

I am surrounded by a team of climbers and mountain guides, who I hope see me as a competent climber, someone who will go on to tackle even harder peaks. They know that I'm adventurous and steadfast, the only woman who signed up for the expedition, keeping pace with the men and refusing to quit. They've learned that I can haul a heavy pack, sleep in the snow, and go without a shower or washing my face for three days, just like the rest of them. I can be just as gritty as the guys, especially in pursuit of the sports I love. I'm not your typical "girl," or your typical neurologist, for that matter.

The details I've chosen to divulge about myself—how long I've been married, where I practice neurology, my favorite places to travel—reflect who I am today. But the other climbers don't know about the darker side of my past. The curved flower tattoo on my left calf, hidden under thermals, soft-shell pants, and merino wool socks, is the symbol for an eating disorder survivor. It's the physical manifestation of an invisible scar that has been with me for years. At the summit, they don't know that the tears pricking the corners of my eyes are tears of happiness and a feeling of accomplishment about how far I've come, rather than from the wind and cold biting at my exposed face.

I visualize my former self: a frail girl in her teens and then twenties who got lost and withered away, physically and emotionally, from anorexia and bulimia. She looks utterly miserable, striving hard to be perfect but never getting there. She learned the hard way that perfection is unattainable, and unnecessary. Happiness was never going to be found in a size 0.

For years, I have carried the ghost of that girl with me on hiking trips, road marathons, and trail ultramarathons. Now I carry her to the top of the mountain. Sometimes she is a voice of strength, a whisper of encouragement that motivates me to keep moving; other times she is an echo of self-doubt and fear of failure, a reminder of how weak I once was. Every physical challenge or endurance race I have completed has been vindication for the 100-pound girl who couldn't muster the strength to run a mile. Every energy gel and nutritious meal I have eaten has been to fuel my muscles and to make up for the hunger she endured. It's time to leave the ghost behind, and the top of Mount Rainier seems like a beautiful final resting place.

I am no longer that girl. I am a strong, successful, ambitious woman. My body fits in a size 8 and is a powerhouse on the trail. Years after my recovery, I have knowledge and insight into my mental illness far beyond anything I learned in medical school or residency—an insight that needs to be shared so that others can avoid the path I traveled. I am a neurologist who has examined her own mind.

I now realize that I was a victim of genetics and environment, that my brain changed with the state of my disease and formed habits that made me feel powerless against it, and that none of it was my fault. By extinguishing unhealthy habits and addictions and finding healthy ones—especially running—I

INTRODUCTION

was able to escape the prison of mental illness, find my true self again, and forgive sixteen-year-old me, who dieted in a desperate attempt to gain control during a turbulent time when she didn't know any better. On the mountain, I am surrounded by the two most powerful therapies I've found, the very things that saved me: exercise and nature.

I start back down the narrow crystalline path of snow and ice that flanks the volcano and listen to the steady crunch of my crampons. I match my breathing to the cadence of my steps, and I feel at peace. The sky is set afire by the rising sun, the path before me illuminated by its rays. I have another ten hours of hiking to return to the trailhead, and beyond that, years of adventures ahead of me. My body is prepared for whatever challenge comes its way.

I battled a severe eating disorder for fourteen years; it took another seven years to call myself recovered. By discovering endurance sports and embracing nature, I overcame my eating disorder in an unconventional way, but one that has led me to achieve great things as an athlete. It is a constant reminder of my willpower and perseverance. I am only beginning to see my own strength, and that realization is enough to carry me back down the mountain.

Chapter 1

LITTLE MISS PERFECT

The night I scored the game-winning goal, it was late autumn, and the air was crisp and cool enough for the fans and parents in the bleachers to bundle up in jackets and sweaters. For us athletes on the field, constant sprinting, pivoting, and vigilant waiting on our toes kept us warm in shorts and short-sleeved jerseys. The floodlights over the soccer field illuminated the nonstop action. I jogged up and down the left side of the field like a panther stalking its prey, waiting for a chance to capture the ball and score for our team. We were in the semifinals for the girls' varsity soccer championship, and the outcome of the game would decide our fate for the rest of the season. The score was tied, with just a sliver of the second half left to go.

The center midfielder kicked the ball hard up the left wing, and I could hear my coach's voice cut like glass through the cheering crowd: "Cait—*GO!*"

The ball landed at my feet, and I leapt into action, tearing down the field as fast as my muscles would take me. I raced past two defenders on a breakaway toward the goal. I planted my right foot and struck the ball as hard as I could with my left, leaning back to angle the shot. I blinked and a moment later saw the ball rocket past the goalkeeper and firmly hit the back of the net. The crowd roared as my teammates clobbered me on the field with hugs and pats on the back. I couldn't stop smiling as we jogged back to the 50-yard line to restart the game. We were just a few minutes from victory.

As I tried to focus on the speech I was giving as salutatorian, my best memories of playing varsity soccer flooded my mind. I missed the cool breeze and excited energy that came with fall soccer games under the lights. It was high school graduation night, and beads of sweat formed under my cap and gown from a combination of nerves and the humid June weather. I was standing on the same football field where I had played most of my soccer games the past four years, the school's only official 100-yard field, where all the major athletic events, pep rallies, parades, and ceremonies were held. Despite a small graduating class of 150 students, there were still enough family members and friends in the bleachers to remind me how much I feared public speaking. Their attentive stares made me choke on my words as if swallowing a handful of cotton balls. And I was sweating, something my body rarely did anymore. I was thin—so thin I felt perpetually cold, even under heavy blankets and sweaters.

Giving a joint speech with the valedictorian alleviated my fear somewhat, and we took turns at the microphone, doling out proverbs and words of encouragement to our classmates. "Keep your head in the game and your eyes on the prize," I said with forced enthusiasm. I didn't truly think my words would impact anyone's future. I was also bitter about not being the

1 | LITTLE MISS PERFECT

valedictorian of my class. Most people defined me by my shining academic career, and my high school graduation book was stamped with the superlative "Class Brains" next to my photo. I came in second at the finish line, and that hurt, but regardless, I would have preferred to be remembered for my athletic achievements, especially since they were fading away as I left for college. I had no idea how much I would come to miss that soccer field in the years that followed.

I grew up in Blairstown, New Jersey, a rural town nestled in the Appalachian Mountains, bordered by the Delaware Water Gap to the west. Blairstown was what most people imagine when they think of small-town life, and the opposite of what they imagine when they think of New Jersey. My hometown had an abundance of farmland and gossip, things that were of little interest to the bored teenagers who loitered in the parking lot after school with nothing else to do. While the town lacked excitement, it also lacked the unsavory things that come with growing up in a city, like crime and overcrowding; the only traffic jams were due to cows wandering across country roads or the Fourth of July parade that spilled across Main Street.

It was a quiet, sheltered place to grow up with my older brother and younger sister, and I was happy playing in the backyard and swinging from the branches of the rhododendron trees that grew in clusters on our three-acre property. Trips to town for errands often involved a stop at the Dairy Queen or the local airport diner for a takeout container of thick, salty french fries. One traffic light guided us to the public library, the gas station, and the grocery store. Blairstown was the middle of nowhere—and the center of my universe. I was the middle child in a cookie-cutter working-class family of five. My dad was a mold maker by trade, at a time when college degrees weren't necessary to earn a middle-class income, and my mom was a housewife by choice, happily staying home to raise the three of us kids. Our two-story Colonial had a big backyard, and behind it stood the Appalachian range, a permanent backdrop of deciduous trees that changed colors from forest green to brick red and burnt caramel every fall.

Nature wove its way into the tapestry of everyday life in Blairstown, something I took for granted and did not fully appreciate until I was an adult living in a city. Nature was there when my brother, sister, and I built snow forts during winter storms, when we ran through the woods playing manhunt as teenagers, when we kicked up piles of crunchy, fragrant leaves while trick-or-treating in the neighborhood. It taught us how to be artists, making sculptures out of mud, painting rocks, and arranging bouquets of dandelions. Most of our time was spent outdoors biking, hiking, and exploring due to the proximity of our house to the Appalachian Trail and an uninhabited Scout camp up the road, which offered plenty of opportunities for adventure. Canoeing and camping out under the stars were staples of summer, when the long sweltering days seemed endless and school was a distant worry.

While Blairstown seemed idyllic to me as a child, I always knew I would outgrow it. Maybe it was overhearing cautionary words from adults, or seeing the same people cycle from the only gas station to the only supermarket to the only bar in town on repeat, but I learned that the town had a gravitational pull that kept its locals inert. High school graduates married their classmates and stayed, creating the next generation that would keep the town population constantly hovering around five thousand. The "townies" who lingered in Blairstown after high school had

1 | LITTLE MISS PERFECT

few opportunities. My brother, Steve, nicknamed it "the place where dreams go to die," and as his gullible little sister, I believed everything he said, even when he tricked me into thinking I was adopted or told me my feet were big enough to fit in clown shoes. If I wanted to escape small-town life, if I wanted to achieve something greater, I had to apply myself in school and go away to college. Being a "townie" was not my destiny.

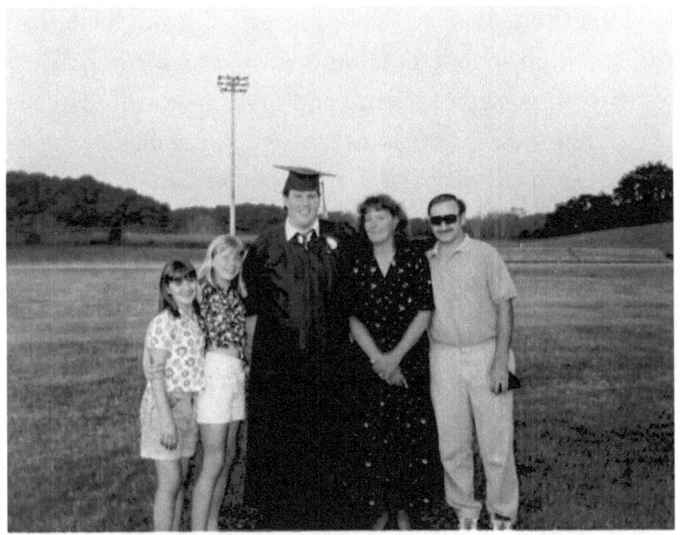

My whole family at Steve's high school graduation

I was naturally smart, a genetic gift from my parents that I sharpened and refined with years of hard work. While other parents were told "She's smart, but she needs to *apply* herself" or "She would do much better if she would sit still and pay attention," my parents could rest assured that I was an excellent student. I was smart; I was diligent; I had *potential*. I listened in class and applied myself while other kids couldn't stop fidgeting. I built science projects and outlined book reports weeks in advance instead of procrastinating until the night before. I memorized vocabulary lists and multiplication tables, took notes with perfect penmanship, and accumulated straight A's and awards for academic excellence.

I took school so seriously that one day in second grade, I lost track of time doing research in the library and got in trouble for skipping class. Who skips class to write a report about saving the manatees when it isn't assigned work? Me. If I was going to be a marine biologist someday, I thought, I had better get to work saving the manatees. As I progressed through elementary, middle, and high school, I maintained that fervor, balancing AP classes with after-school science and math meets, all while vying to have the highest grade point average in my class.

I was a perfectionist and a rule follower, the quintessential "goody-goody," the teacher's pet. I couldn't help it; it was ingrained in me to do well. I liked finishing first, collecting blue ribbons and flawless report cards. Some kids at school found it annoying; others were jealous. Even my best friends tired of my achievements, nicknaming me "Little Miss Perfect." Other kids didn't celebrate perfection the way teachers and parents did. Collectively, those kids saw my strengths and chose to focus on my weaknesses, to drag me down from my pedestal.

I was picked on for being a nerd and ostracized by the popular kids in school. Being nearsighted and having acne were flaws that other kids could poke fun at, minor imperfections that made me a target for teasing. When I permed my hair and it came out frizzy, looking more like crinkle cut fries than lustrous curls, they ambushed me. The first to raise my hand in class but the last to defend myself, I quietly let them chip away at my veneer. I was a social pariah. My only redeeming quality, in the eyes of my peers, was that I was also a jock.

---

1 | LITTLE MISS PERFECT

Unlike earning straight A's, being an athlete was relatable, even likeable. A varsity jacket was coveted, even when it belonged to a dorky freshman with ruler-straight bangs and glasses. I gravitated toward soccer from an early age, playing on recreational teams from the age of five. My parents chose the sport for me, but I grew to love it as if I had handpicked it myself. Even as a child, my legs were built for sprinting and darting across the soccer field, with the strength, stability, and balance to plant with one leg and kick with the other. My arms were uncoordinated—too clumsy to dribble a basketball, too weak to pitch a baseball—but I didn't need strong arms to play soccer, and I quickly realized where I belonged.

I was lucky to be entering sports at a time when girls were encouraged as athletes. Thanks to Title IX, growing up in the 1990s meant there was a whole new world of organized sports for female athletes. We didn't have to play one sport; we could choose from a full menu. But for girls who excelled in a sport at a young age, competitive options were still limited, especially in Blairstown. By the age of nine, I was ready to move beyond the recreational soccer field to greener grass.

I tried out for the boys' traveling soccer team, my first chance to break through the confines of small-town life, and I made it. With every away game, I ran the lengths of faraway soccer fields, on grass that seemed as foreign as a new country beneath my feet. It felt adventurous and exciting. Being the only girl on the team wasn't so bad, except for the awkward moments when I changed in and out of my jersey, twisting my arms into a pretzel to avoid exposing my skin, while the boys casually took their shirts off. That inconvenience was easily forgotten when I got to start the game as left striker.

"Way to go, Emmitt!" my dad called from the sidelines. Playing soccer with the boys seemed to earn respect from my dad, enough so that he nicknamed his blonde, fair-skinned daughter after a burly NFL running back. I wanted to please my parents and make them proud, so I took the nickname and ran with it, even though I would have preferred to be compared to my soccer idol, Mia Hamm. Together, my parents were stern but loving; they valued a strong work ethic. But they never pressured me to perform academically or in sports; the drive to succeed came from within, and I strived to be their golden child. In the face of failure, of not being good enough, I punished myself before they had the chance to do so, and forced myself to do better the next time.

It wasn't hard to impress my mom—she marveled at everything my siblings and I did, with words of encouragement and hugs as warm as the freshly baked brownies that greeted us when we got home from school. Being a mom was her greatest joy in life, and she relished every minute of it. She was a constant cheerleader at the sidelines, watching soccer games, attending band recitals, and collecting certificates, newspaper clippings, and artwork in scrapbooks to memorialize everything we did. Her motto, "A winner never quits, and a quitter never wins," lingered in the back of my mind with every endeavor I took on.

My dad, on the other hand, was much harder to impress. He didn't dole out praise regularly, so when he did, it felt like winning a carnival game, with the fanfare of flashing lights and ringing bells and jealous siblings looking on. He was a jack-of-all-trades when it came to sports, a sturdily built man who dabbled in everything from downhill skiing and mountain biking to running and dirt bike racing. What impressed him most was athletic performance, and it was obvious to my brother, sister, and me that he enjoyed coaching and watching our games far more than he enjoyed picking apples or helping with homework. I inherited his stocky Polish thighs and knack for sport—one more point in favor of the golden child.

1 | LITTLE MISS PERFECT

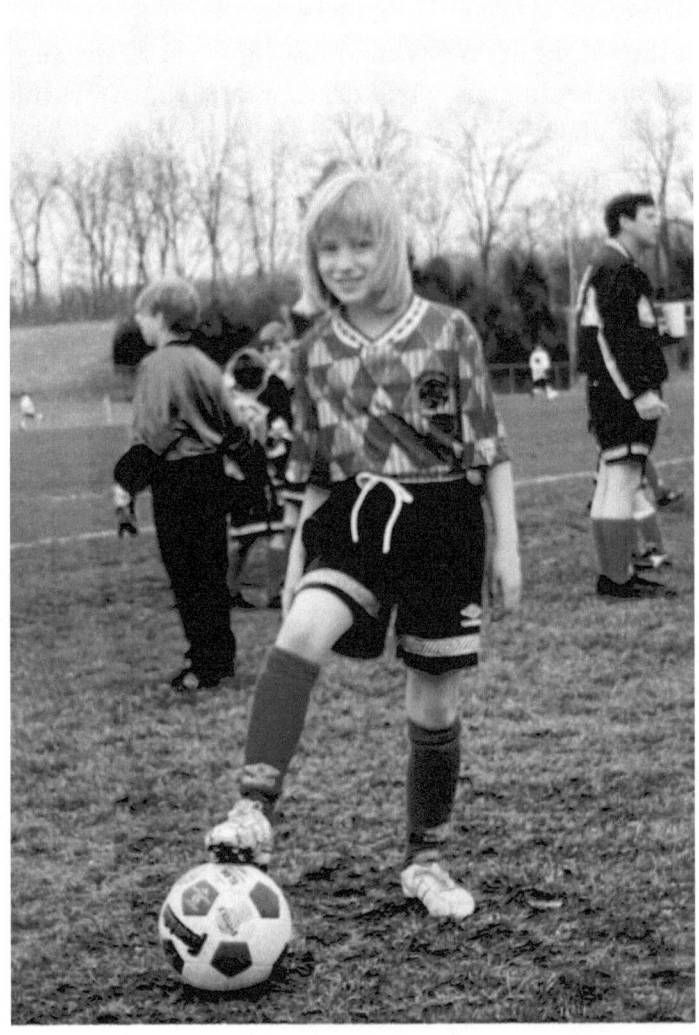

On the boys' soccer team

Then puberty messed everything up. Until that point, my strength had matched that of the boys on the team, and I had no reason to believe I couldn't beat them in a sprint to the ball.

But a surge in testosterone levels made their muscles stronger and leaner, and suddenly I couldn't keep pace. My figure softened with the weight of breasts and fuller hips, and all the angular parts of me became curvy. It felt like I was trading in my athletic ability for a body I wasn't sure I wanted, a body that would slow me down.

I was torn, caught between wanting to be "one of the boys" on the travel team and wanting to be attractive to the boys at school, even the boys on the team. I crushed on my teammates, but to them I was just another pair of cleats with a strong left foot. I asked my mom to buy me a sports bra, to hide the part of me that made me most unlike my teammates, so I could belong a little while longer. But a bra was just a padded Band-Aid; I couldn't cover the fact that I was growing into a young woman. My time on the boys' team had reached its end.

When I joined the girls' soccer team at my school, I was surrounded by teammates who were facing the same insecurities, and on the girls' team, I didn't have to sneak tampons into my pocket or hide in a bathroom stall to change my shirt. I could be a teenage girl, uncomfortable in my body, just like everyone else around me. I could be shy, reserved, and unpopular, but somehow still fit in. And I could still be a good soccer player. When I started my freshman year of high school on the JV team and was quickly promoted to varsity, I realized I could be great.

It was tradition to meet at someone's house or an Italian restaurant the night before a big game, where we would eat with reckless abandon, soaking up as many carbohydrates as possible to fuel us for the next day. Alisa, blonde-haired and Polish like me, was a center midfielder whose mom regularly opened up her home and her kitchen. Every few weeks, we gathered around their dinner table, where heaping bowls of pasta with red sauce, garlic bread, meatballs, and Caesar salad were passed around in a frenzy of hands and utensils. Calorie-oblivious eating was part of the experience of playing on the team—as were the endless summer camps, double training sessions, and long after-school practices. Being on the team could be a grueling commitment, but I loved it.

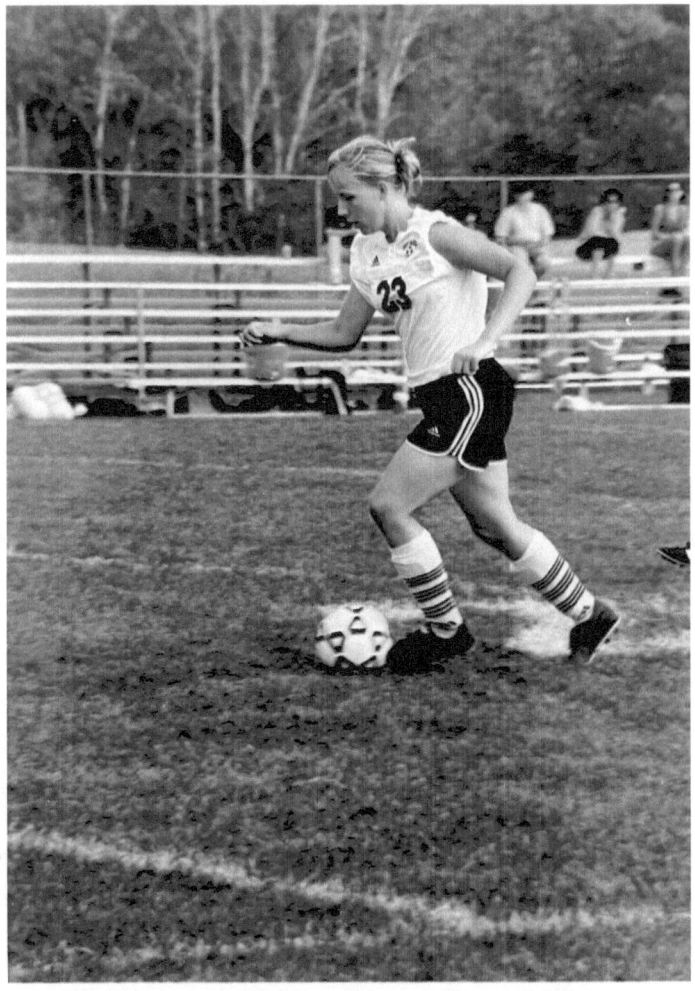

On the varsity soccer team

My body was made for soccer, with strong calves and quads and the ability to fly down the field at a breakneck pace. My lungs were able to keep up, and I rarely felt out of breath. Even though I was teased for my "thunder thighs" and "bubble butt" and jeans never seemed to fit right, I realized being muscular wasn't a bad thing. My solidly built legs allowed me to outrun defenders and sprint to the opponent's goal. When we underperformed in practice or a game, and our coach punished us with 100-yard sprints on repeat, I ran with a vengeance, beating my teammates to the goalpost at the opposite end of the field. Seventeen seconds of hard sprinting—only to do it again and again.

I was constantly running—running for the ball, running to score a goal, running to warm up for a game, running fartleks and hill sprints during drills. I was fast enough to be on the track team, if our school would ever build a track. And yet I never considered myself a runner. I was a soccer player, and that was all I needed to keep me fit and happy. I was surrounded by a group of energetic, like-minded girls who loved the game too. I didn't have to look in a mirror to see my reflection; their bodies looked just like mine, muscular and sturdy, and I felt like I belonged. Once my sister, Kerin, started high school and took the position of left midfielder, a slide-tackling force behind me on the field, the team felt complete.

My life was a contented routine of school, soccer, and sleep, punctuated by weekends of lazing about the house with my family, eating bacon-and-egg sandwiches at the kitchen table while we traded the sports and comic pages of the Sunday morning newspaper. I had found my niche in the world. It was predictable, but to me, predictable was comforting. Chaos and uncertainty gave me butterflies. As a perfectionist, I liked everything to be neat, organized, and safely tucked into place; my room was spotlessly clean, my closet a color-coded system of hanging clothes.

1 | LITTLE MISS PERFECT

Schoolbooks and folders were stacked with precision on my desk, Post-it tabs sticking out at perfect right angles so I knew where to find what I needed. I had it all figured out. For a teenager, I was composed, on top of my game, in control. I was a varsity soccer player and a model student. Any deviation from perfection caused anxiety, and I worked hard to keep things exactly the way I liked them. So if an unmade bed or dirty dish unraveled me, it was no surprise that my parents' divorce completely upended my world.

Chapter 2

PERFECT STORM

"Dad is leaving," my mom said. He was there one day and gone the next. When he left, the pickup truck bed was empty, as if he were going out for milk or running an errand at the hardware store. It was snowing that late spring day near the end of my sophomore year. I peered out my bedroom window at the contrast of the drifting snowflakes against the blossoming trees and contemplated the disappearance of someone who had been a stabilizing force in my life. Everything blurred, a milkshake of green and white beyond the glass windowpane. Had he even said goodbye?

As a teenager, living in my own egocentric bubble, I didn't pay much attention to family dynamics. It was normal to fight with my sister over the shared phone line, and for my mom to quarrel with my sister when she was running late for school. If my brother locked his door and blasted Nirvana through the stereo, we knew to keep out. When my parents argued, they tucked away behind the closed door of their bedroom and kept it muted; we never bothered to eavesdrop. There were plenty of times we coexisted peacefully and even enjoyed each other's company. But in the months leading up to my dad's departure, there was a gradual, palpable buildup of tension in the house, and it thickened the air like a churning, rolling thunderhead before a storm; my sister and I felt it, unsure whether to confront it or retreat and hide in our rooms. One day the storm cloud broke and released its destruction—my parents were getting divorced.

Don't cry, I told myself, as I watched his truck roll away down the snow-dusted road. Even though I wasn't close with my dad, I didn't want him to leave; he was Dad, a permanent fixture in my life, a fact as true as the earth is round. I didn't break down in tears, but an uneasy sadness washed over me. Troubling, unanswered questions bounced around inside my head. *Why did he leave? Would he ever come back? Was it something I did? Were we not good enough?* These were questions I couldn't voice aloud—I was too afraid to know the truth, too young and naive to meddle in my parents' relationship—so I let them ping-pong back and forth in my mind.

In a family that hated yelling and embraced quiet at the dinner table, my siblings and I were raised to be stoic, to never wear our emotions on our sleeves. We were taught to internalize our feelings and hold back our tears, so that is exactly what we did when my father left: We soldiered on. But my dad was the breadwinner in our household, and without him, everything slowly fell apart. My mom was devastated. She had put all her faith into twenty-five years of marriage, and when that marriage failed, there was no college degree or career path to fall back on. She tried to make ends meet by cleaning houses and working odd jobs, collecting handfuls of twenty-dollar bills under the table, but without a steady income, she spent her days on her hands and knees, scrubbing toilets and struggling to keep the fridge stocked.

Kerin and I sat at the kitchen table one night, clipping grocery store coupons and looking up recipes for dinner while my mom worked late. The last working lightbulb flickered overhead and then fizzled out. I couldn't remember the last time we had spent money on something as trivial as lightbulbs. "What about this recipe?" I asked. "We can make a tuna noodle casserole and crush up corn flakes to bake on top as the crust. We have all the ingredients." It looked completely unappetizing, but we made it anyway and saved the leftovers for my mom. Gloppy beige filling bubbled up through the cracks of corn flake crust. I was proud of our creation. We became experts at creating meals with whatever we could find in the house, but after a while, the monotony of white rice, canned vegetables, and cereal left a sour taste in my mouth.

After my dad left, I mourned not only the loss of our family but also the loss of all the luxuries I had been used to. I said goodbye to my mom's home-cooked meals, as she had neither the time to make them nor the money to buy the ingredients. Gone were dinners out and shopping trips for school clothes, things that felt viscerally painful to a teenager but probably seemed frivolous to an adult. I didn't *need* those things to survive, but I wanted them. It seemed as though we had gone from being a functional middle-class family to one that was broken and poverty-stricken overnight.

I envied my older brother, Steve, who had moved out by that time, distanced from the wreckage. He would always remember our home when it was full of life and happiness and family dinners, when my dad's salary kept the pantry stocked and the utilities running. He didn't have to see the house falling into disrepair, the dust accumulating on the gingham kitchen curtains, the broken washing machine, or the dish detergent bottle filled with water to eke out the last few drops of soap.

I looked to my mom as the last pillar of strength that would keep our household erect. She had always been the heart of our home, radiating warmth and reassurance that everything would be okay. She was the one who bandaged scraped knees, kissed foreheads when they burned with fever, and comforted us after nightmares. She was also hardworking, diligently cleaning as many houses as she could each week in order to pay the mortgage. Her hands, like her gentle soul, wore thin with the effort of constant scrubbing, wiping, and dusting, and her clothes smelled faintly of Windex and lemon Pledge by the end of each day.

During spring and summer breaks, I cleaned houses with her. It was backbreaking work, spending all day bent over a vacuum cleaner, scrubbing dirty toilets and showers, and picking away at grimy kitchen counters with steel wool sponges until sweat permeated my T-shirt and calluses formed on my palms. My mom never stopped moving, even when the bored, rich housewives in their nightgowns followed her around chatting and sipping their coffee. They had nowhere to be, but she was motivated to finish the job, collect her pay, and move on to the next house. When she offered me cash, I turned it down—the stack of crisp green bills was enticing, but I didn't have the heart to take it from her.

After work, Kerin and I watched her retreat into her room, hoping the peace and quiet of being left alone for ten minutes would provide her some solace after a day of arduous labor. But she was emotionally and physically exhausted, and despite our best efforts, she spiraled deeper into depression and turned to alcohol to cope. Empty vodka bottles formed a line under the kitchen sink, a tally of her pain. All we could offer her as consolation was lukewarm tuna noodle casserole.

When Mom told us to pack our bags for summer vacation, I was thrilled. A vacation was a sign of hope, of the normalcy that

I longed for. Every year our family had driven to Ocean City, Maryland, for a weeklong beach vacation. Just hearing the word "beach" evoked memories of building sandcastles, boogieboarding with my dad, running to the ice cream truck for melting strawberry shortcake bars, and smelling the salty ocean breeze. The beach was our family oasis. My suitcase was packed neatly with stacks of T-shirts, Umbro shorts, and bathing suits for the trip, with flip-flops and ten-dollar sunglasses perched on top. I couldn't wait to bury my feet in the sand and stare out at the blurry line where the waves meet the sky.

Then, the day before the trip, my mom gave Kerin and me the bad news. "Sorry, girls. We won't be able to go this year. The condo we usually stay at had a fire, and our place got burned." It was a white lie, designed to hide an ugly truth: There was no vacation. There was no fire. We simply couldn't afford it. I felt gullible and stupid, like I had fallen for a prank, and my excitement turned into anger. I was angry at my mom for lying to me, angry at my dad for leaving us destitute, and angry at the world because I was sixteen. I quietly unpacked my suitcase and buried my clothes and my feelings back in the dresser drawers.

Just like my mom, I became depressed and anxious. I didn't need a professional to diagnose me, and we couldn't have afforded one anyway. My only escape was to throw on my raggedy old sneakers and run up and down the road. One mile out, one mile back. Running was hard when there was no soccer goal or sideline to focus on, but it became a bit easier every time I did it. The road was flat and ran parallel to the Appalachian Mountains, a beautiful place to lose track of time, stare out at the trees, and distract myself from the reality of everyday life. It gave me peace. I didn't realize it at the time, but running outside was the most calming therapy I would find, and it would become a huge part of my life later on.

Even as the seasons changed and the temperature dropped to a frigid 20°F in January, I bundled up in a sweatshirt and mittens, letting my exposed ears and nose feel the sting of the air as I jogged. Everything was barren and gray, and it hurt to breathe in the icy air, but the harsh winter weather felt good. It made me feel alive at a time when the depressed mood inside the house, and inside my own mind, seemed to rob me of sensation.

Sometimes I listened to music or the sound of my feet hitting the pavement; other times I ruminated about how life had taken a turn for the worse. I wondered if I was partly to blame for my dad's disappearance. I had tried so hard to be the golden child, the high achiever, the award-winning athlete and student—but what if that wasn't enough? How could I have been better? Sometimes my thoughts turned dark and angry, and my pace quickened. How could he leave my mom like this? We were uninsured. Where the fuck was the child support payment when I needed a cavity filled? Was he out there somewhere eating filet mignon while we ate stewed tomatoes and rice for dinner? I was spinning. My teenage brain started looking for other ways to regain control, to recreate the perfect life I missed.

When I lost the first few pounds, it was by accident. School days were followed by two-hour soccer practices and part-time shifts at Dale's Market, the local deli where I learned every brand of cigarette and chewing tobacco and stacked them in alphabetical order behind the counter to sell to the townies. I barely had time to think about food. With less food in the house and a busy schedule, five pounds magically melted away. *If I could lose five pounds without trying*, I thought, *I wonder how much I could lose with a little effort.* That was when I decided to diet.

It started slowly, eliminating foods that seemed to be obviously bad for me, like french fries and cookies—foods that most people could benefit from reducing in their diet. Then we got rid of meat, a way to lower the grocery bill disguised as an ethical stance against animal cruelty. The scarcity of food in the house forced me to eat mostly processed foods, frozen and packaged junk foods that were cheaper than fresh fruits and vegetables, so I became picky and ate the ones that were lowest in calories.

It felt good to get rid of things in my diet, a sort of cleanse not unlike spring cleaning or shredding old papers. It felt like starting over. But instead of getting rid of trash, I was throwing out entire food groups. I was still playing soccer every day, burning through every calorie I ate, so even small changes to my diet made a huge difference. Over a few months, my weight dropped from 140 to 126 pounds, and I felt *amazing*! My size 10 jeans hung loosely on my hips. "You look so *skinny*," my friends said. "You're so *thin* now!" No one had ever called me that before.

I soaked up the compliments greedily; they were positive reinforcement, a reason to keep losing weight. If I kept dieting, maybe all the teasing about my thunder thighs would go away. Maybe boys would notice me and ask me out. I would store away the confidence and self-assurance that came with being admired and take it with me when I left for college. Having control over what I ate gave me a renewed sense of achievement, and that was even more rewarding than the weight loss itself.

Kerin and I leafed through the racks at H&M, arms weighed down with clothes as we headed toward the dressing room. We couldn't afford them, but trying on a dozen outfits and modeling them for each other was a good way to pass a boring, rainy afternoon. I stood in my bra and underwear and studied my new profile in the dressing room mirror. The layer of baby fat that had hugged my upper thighs and hips was gone, and my stomach was as flat as a pancake. I sucked in my breath, eyeing the faint outline of my ribs through the stretchy V-neck shirt I had on. I felt thin*er* and prett*ier*, but I could do better.

When I was done trying on clothes, I shoved a few bras and T-shirts without ink tags into my bag and buried them beneath my notebook and makeup. My heart fluttered like a hummingbird. As I walked through the threshold of the store and back out into the mall without making a purchase, I was hit with a rush of adrenaline. I had gotten away with it again. We had no money to buy new clothes, and nothing in my closet fit anymore. I knew shoplifting was a dishonest, risky thing to do—it was the opposite of what Little Miss Perfect would do—but now I was the poor girl who couldn't go shopping because her dad didn't make his child support payments. It wasn't fair. The world had wronged me, so what did it matter if I perpetuated the wrongdoing?

The dieting continued through my junior and senior years of high school, and my weight steadily dropped—to 115 pounds and then to 110 pounds. Somehow, despite my progress, I never felt thin enough. The overachiever in me took it as a challenge to see how many more pounds I could shed. I kept track of how long I could make it through the day without eating anything. It was a punishing game—leaving for school without breakfast, resisting the greasy pizza and warm chocolate chip cookies in the cafeteria at lunch, and waiting to have a snack until I put on my shin guards and cleats before soccer practice. No one knew why I was biting into an apple or granola bar as savagely as a hyena might dig into the carcass of its prey. It was just enough to keep me on my feet during practice.

2 | PERFECT STORM

With the cash I made from my part-time job, I bought a cheap, shiny white scale from Wal-Mart and tracked my weight diligently at home. I weighed myself every morning, anxiously willing my weight to be less than the day before. Every day was a turn at the slot machine, as I waited for the blinking numbers to solidify in front of my toes. Would I be rewarded with a number that was one pound, two pounds less? Would I be disappointed when the number hadn't budged? The unpredictability of the scale kept me coming back for more, fiending for an intangible reward. Perfection was quantifiable, the same way it had been when I earned 100 on a test, but now it was measured by the number of calories I ate and the number of pounds on the scale.

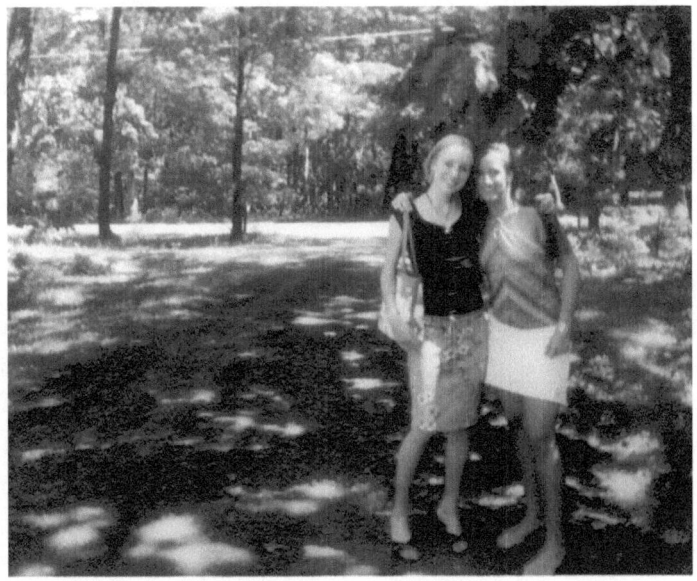

With my sister, Kerin (one of the few photos of me with anorexia)

"Maybe you should talk to someone," my mom suggested, looking concerned. We were sitting at an award luncheon with other soccer players and their parents. It wasn't the award that made that day special; it was that my mom and I got to spend a day out, dressed up and enjoying a catered lunch without worrying about the bill. She wore a dress and heels and had styled her hair for the occasion. A delicious meal of pasta with Alfredo sauce, chicken, garlic bread, and salad was spread across the white linen tablecloth as the award ceremony began. It was just like the meals Alisa's mom made before games, but I no longer wanted it. I could barely stomach a diet soda and a few bites of salad. Moving my fork toward the pile of creamy pasta on my plate was like putting my hand into a terrarium of hissing snakes. I inched away from the table, fearful that every calorie I ate would make me gain weight. I wanted to run out of the banquet hall and keep running as far away from food as I could get.

After the luncheon, stomach growling from my refusal to eat, I nibbled on a package of crackers in the car. I pulled each peanut butter cracker sandwich apart, savoring one half and then the other to make the package last longer. "I'm sorry, Mom," I said. "I didn't mean to be so cranky. But I feel better now." She looked sad and worried, and that made me feel even worse. I had fucked up our special day, and the guilt was crushing me beneath my seatbelt.

One of my teammates' mothers had alerted my mom that I looked "sick." As I would learn later, there were many reasons my mother hadn't noticed my drastic weight loss, but once she saw it, she couldn't unsee it. She let it go that day, but I ended up in the offices of the guidance counselor and school nurse later that month. "I'm fine," I assured them. "I'm just trying to eat healthy, and I play soccer a *lot*. I can't help it if I've lost a few pounds." I was cutting out the truth as readily as I was cutting out calories. All I wanted was for them to stop scrutinizing me, and my excuses seemed to work.

Once the concerned adults in my life let me be, I breathed a sigh of relief at being invisible again. I had shrunk from a size 10 to a size 0, and I was proud of my progress. But the compliments had gone away. When I passed my friends and peers in the hallway, I sometimes felt their sideways glances. Others chose to look away completely, as if I had a disease that might be contagious. But I didn't *feel* sick; I felt successful in my mission to become skinny.

While the weight loss temporarily improved my speed on the soccer field, I was losing muscle mass and power, and that led to a gradual decline in my performance level. By senior year, I was sluggish during drills and slow to sprint to the ball, but I dug in harder to compensate and remained a valuable player on the team. I stopped getting my period, but not having it actually made my teenage life easier. The only thing that never seemed to get better was my mood. I thought that losing weight would make me happy, but I was still depressed, and even more anxious than when I had started.

I was unaware of the destruction that was occurring beneath the surface of my skin. Years later in medical school, I would learn that I was starving not only my muscles but also my hypothalamus, a part of the brain that plays a crucial role in stimulating the pituitary gland and regulating sex hormones. That triggered a cascade of hormonal changes in my body, leading to amenorrhea, or absent menstrual periods, bone loss, muscle loss, and low energy. And depression, triggered by my parents' divorce, was amplified by the weight loss, yet another symptom of my starving brain.

It is unclear exactly when I became anorexic. I traced it back to the day my dad drove off in his truck, the day that caused a fissure in the foundation of our family. But in reality, it took a long time to develop this severe mental health disorder. By definition, it would have been when my body mass index (BMI), or ratio of body weight to height, fell below 18.5, the lower limit of "normal." According to the most recent edition of the *Diagnostic and Statistical Manual of Mental Disorders*, Fifth Edition, commonly referred to as the DSM-5, anorexia nervosa is defined as:

A. Restriction of energy intake relative to requirements, leading to a significantly low body weight in the context of age, sex, developmental trajectory, and physical health. Significantly low body weight is a weight that is less than minimally normal or, for children and adolescents, less than that minimally expected.
B. Intense fear of gaining weight or becoming fat or persistent behavior that interferes with weight gain, even though at a significantly low weight.
C. Disturbance in the way in which one's body weight or shape is experienced, undue influence of body weight or shape on self-evaluation, or persistent lack of recognition of current low body weight.

I checked all these boxes and then some. I went from healthy to thin to underweight. I became a walking nutritional index, able to rattle off the caloric content and serving size of everything from oatmeal to a hard-boiled egg. Everything was measured in tablespoons, ounces, and half cups. While everyone else filled their plate, I restricted myself to portioned low-calorie foods, gulping down water and diet soda to trick my stomach into feeling full. I even turned down Thanksgiving dinner, loading my plate with steamed broccoli and avoiding the mashed potatoes and casseroles that made my mouth water. When my family urged me to try the cranberry sauce and pumpkin pie, I said no, too stubborn in my resolve to be "healthy," too fearful of the consequences of eating such delicious food.

I never told my soccer coach or my mom, the two trustworthy female figures in my life, that I had lost my period. Maybe if I had, they would have forced me to quit the soccer team and focus on my health. Or maybe they would have sent me to talk to a therapist or a nutritionist. As a soccer player, I wasn't supposed to have an eating disorder. I was on a team of healthy, strong young women, each with her own unique strengths on the soccer field. There was no value in being thinner than the next girl.

Playing sports didn't drive my obsession with being thin; my anorexia was fueled by factors that I couldn't control and that I would only come to understand years later. And in the end, sports would come back to save me from myself.

Chapter 3

NATURE + NURTURE + STRESS

Destiny is a predetermined course of events that arises from an irresistible force—a hidden, sometimes magical power that controls what will happen in the future. We refer to destiny every day, crediting positive outcomes to good luck, fortune, and serendipity, and blaming negative events on doom or fate. We use it to explain why we are the way we are, why we end up married, alone, successful, unemployed, happy, discontent.

Science has its own version of destiny, and it is based on the inheritable, biological, and environmental factors that shape who we are. It's called "nature versus nurture," and it's been around since behavioral geneticist Francis Galton popularized the concept in the late 1800s. It is the idea that, as adults, our traits are the product of either our genes or our environment from the time we are born. Nature and nurture are not mutually exclusive though; they can work synergistically, sometimes in our favor, other times against us.

In someone who is predisposed to psychological illness by way of nature and nurture, adding an acute stressor to the mix can catalyze the development of a mental health crisis. In the field of psychology, this is known as the diathesis-stress model. For example, when a person is born into a family with a strong history of alcoholism (nature), is surrounded by parents and relatives who are constantly drinking (nurture), and later marries someone who enjoys binge drinking, getting fired from their job (an acute stressor) might provoke them to hit the bar, drink themselves into oblivion, and come back the next day to do it all over again, sparking a serious alcohol addiction. For me, the equation was:

Nature + nurture + the destruction of my family = eating disorder

Was I not mentally tough enough to deal with the stressors that were thrown at me as a teenager? Was my eating disorder a choice? Or was my brain just *wired* for mental illness? When I was anorexic and later bulimic, I believed it was my destiny to be held hostage by my eating disorder for the rest of my life, that there was no escape, that it was my penance for choosing to diet in the first place. When nature versus nurture was taught over and over in biology courses throughout high school, college, and then medical school, it went in one ear and out the other. I could never apply it to my own life, to sort out why I was the way I was. I was too busy sinking in the quicksand of my eating disorder. Only years after my recovery could I look back and examine the ways my mind went astray.

Eating disorders, in the form of anorexia nervosa, bulimia nervosa, and binge eating disorder, fall along a spectrum of neuropsychiatric disorders that manifest as dysregulation of appetite, weight, and behavioral changes related to eating. According to the National Eating Disorders Association, more than twenty-eight million Americans will experience an eating disorder at some point in their lives.[1] This equates to a lifetime prevalence of 1 percent for anorexia nervosa, 1 to 2 percent for bulimia nervosa, and 3 percent for binge eating disorder, with the disorders being twice as prevalent in females as in males.

Eating disorders are chronic conditions that can lead to severe medical complications, such as dangerous electrolyte imbalances, cardiac arrhythmias, and organ failure due to malnutrition. Far too often, people with eating disorders cycle through medical and psychiatric hospitalizations, no closer to a cure for their illness. Ultimately, some will die. Eating disorders are one of the most lethal of all psychiatric disorders, second only to substance use disorders, with suicide being a leading cause of death.[2] As if having one defined eating disorder isn't punishment enough, many people cross over from one syndrome to another during their protracted illness.

My eating disorder started as anorexia, then shapeshifted into binge eating, and eventually into bingeing and purging, or bulimia. I will later discuss why that happened, and how my brain became addicted to food. But first, there was anorexia, which ruled my life from age sixteen to twenty-one.

Nature

With respect to nature, two fundamental factors are brain development and genetics.

The average age of onset for anorexia nervosa and bulimia nervosa is eighteen. By definition, eighteen is the age at which a person is considered an adult, with the right to vote, make autonomous decisions, and accept full legal responsibility for their actions. In reality, though, the mind of an eighteen-year-old is still malleable, impressionable, and susceptible to external influences that can affect their decision-making capabilities. That is because the brain of an eighteen-year-old is not fully developed. Accordingly, early adulthood is considered to be a vulnerable brain age.

At birth, the brain contains around eighty-six billion neurons, with fifty trillion neural connections, or synapses, communicating between them. That sounds like a lot, until you compare that number to a fully developed adult brain, where the number of synapses is closer to *five hundred* trillion. The process of brain development takes decades rather than years. Myelination—a process that improves the speed of communication between neurons, much like adding insulation or sheathing to electrical wires—is complete in most parts of the brain by age fifteen to seventeen, but some pivotal parts lag behind, particularly in the frontal lobes.

During the adolescent years, behaviors are driven by the limbic system, a complex group of structures involved in emotional regulation and memory. The limbic system is the part of the brain that encourages teenagers to be impulsive and try risky, exciting things—smoking a cigarette, drinking alcohol, having sex. It also plays a pivotal role in habit formation and addiction, the focus of a later chapter as it relates to bulimia. It can take nearly another decade for the frontal lobes to catch up and run as smoothly as the rest of the electrical circuit, to control the on/off switch that keeps the limbic system in check.

The frontal lobes, the brain's largest region, are the most important part of the brain for functioning in the real world and behaving as socially appropriate human beings. They are made up of multiple distinct areas involved in everything from voluntary

3 | NATURE + NURTURE + STRESS

movement to expressive language to the ability to control our bladders. Sitting toward the front of the frontal lobes, the captain of the ship, is the aptly named prefrontal cortex. Some call it the brain's CEO; sports psychologists call it the central governor, a concept we'll discuss later as it relates to endurance running.

The prefrontal cortex makes the rules that dictate how we behave through three main functions: restraint, or the ability to inhibit inappropriate behaviors; initiative, the motivation to pursue activities and be productive; and order, the ability to perform sequencing tasks, abstract reasoning, and planning. When we make a decision, judge a situation, persevere through an obstacle, wait patiently or delay gratification, stay focused, or multi-task—all the things we do daily in our adult lives—we have the prefrontal cortex to thank. The very traits we consider part of our personality, such as patience, kindness, neatness, curiosity, and creativity, stem from this area of the brain.

This part of the brain also steers us away from making bad, impulsive choices; instead of binge drinking or trying cocaine and partying all night, behaviors that are counterproductive to adult life, it tells us to stay home and get enough sleep so we can go to work the next day and collect a paycheck. When the frontal lobes are damaged by an event such as a stroke or brain tumor, the resulting symptoms are unpredictable. Some people become apathetic, while others may be mute, depressed, manic, or even hypersexual. Impairment of frontal lobe function can strip away any semblance of our former self and completely alter our personality. That is, the symptoms impact who we are in the world.

My favorite example of this is the story of Phineas Gage, a railroad construction foreman who suffered a traumatic brain injury. In 1848, he survived a grisly accident in which a large iron rod penetrated his skull and went directly into his left frontal lobe. After the accident, he retained knowledge and memory, but according to his doctor, he went from being a hardworking, capable foreman to someone completely unrecognizable.

> The equilibrium or balance, so to speak, between his intellectual faculties and animal propensities, seems to have been destroyed. He is fitful, irreverent, indulging at times in the grossest profanity (which was not previously his custom), manifesting but little deference for his fellows, impatient of restraint or advice when it conflicts with his desires, at times pertinaciously obstinate . . .[3]

As the first known case looking at the brain's role in personality, his story is now a part of neurology folklore and the curriculum of every medical student.

Phineas may have lost his frontal lobe functions, but I had barely had time to develop mine when my eating disorder struck. When my sixteen-year-old brain decided to diet, my prefrontal cortex didn't have a strong enough voice to tell me not to. I lacked insight into what a diet could lead to and how it would affect the health of my maturing body. I saw only the positive effects of it: increased self-confidence and a smaller number on the scale.

The second factor to consider with respect to nature is genetics. The genetics of eating disorders is not straightforward. Research has shown that there are several genes that modify the risk of developing an eating disorder, but they are in no way a direct cause. In 2017, *The American Journal of Psychiatry* published a study on the genome-wide association of anorexia nervosa that identified several inheritable genetic loci—the physical location of genetic markers—in our chromosomes.[4] These scientific discoveries, while interesting, are not very useful in real life. The parents of a child with anorexia (or suspected anorexia) are more likely to seek out a nutritionist or a psychologist than a geneticist for help. What is more relevant is how genes affect families and how they play a role in personality. Patterns of behavior within individuals and their families can be clues to recognizing someone who is at higher risk of an eating disorder—and possibly preventing it before it begins.

There are strong trends within family, twin, and population studies that support the idea of heritability. If you have a first-degree relative with anorexia, there is an elevenfold risk that you will also develop it; for bulimia, the risk is somewhere between four- and ninefold. These associations are even stronger when looked at in twins, where heritability has a range of 28 to 58 percent and 54 to 83 percent for anorexia and bulimia, respectively.[5] And, as we will discuss later, eating disorders don't happen in isolation. Oftentimes they overlap with addictions and mood disorders, which can cluster in families. In my family of origin, three of the five of us have had eating disorders; my mom was anorexic, and my brother has struggled with binge eating disorder for most of his life. All five of us have had symptoms of mood disorders and anxiety disorders, including depression, anxiety, and panic attacks. Three have had addictions to food, alcohol, or nicotine. I can't help but think that the genetic deck was stacked against us.

The genetics of personality traits is even murkier, but there are undoubtedly traits ingrained in us from birth. As a chunky-legged toddler, I clumsily walked around cleaning up toys and trash off the floor. I liked neatness, order, and organization, while my sister liked to throw her clothes into a messy pile. I can't explain why I'm a neat freak, just like I can't explain why I'm introverted or moody, or why I prefer quiet over noise. It's just who I am.

We know that genes play a role in personality, and certain personality traits are linked to a higher likelihood of developing an eating disorder. The same study that looked at chromosomes in people with anorexia[6] showed a correlation between anorexia, neuroticism, and educational attainment. Rigid black-and-white thinking, perfectionism, and being an overachiever are traits often found in people who experience anorexia. Compulsiveness, novelty seeking, reward seeking, and excessive worry are traits often found in those who experience binge eating disorder or bulimia. But not everyone who likes to travel binges on donuts on the plane, and not every high school valedictorian (or runner-up) develops anorexia. Many people with these higher-risk traits live fulfilling, successful lives without eating disorders ever crossing their radar. That's where nurture comes in.

Nurture

The first time I walked the beach comfortably in a bathing suit, completely uncovered, without a T-shirt or a towel wrapped around me, was at the age of thirty-two. I was waiting for a judgmental look, a whistle, a laugh—anything to draw attention to my exposed body—but no one cared. Because it was *normal* to wear a bathing suit on the beach. I was no longer anorexic or bulimic, no longer ashamed of my body, but I didn't know how to expose my skin in a normal way, whether I was fat or thin or in-between. Covering up was a learned behavior that had stayed with me from childhood, when nurture started layering onto nature.

When my parents were married, we had home-cooked dinners together as a family, and my brother, sister, and I constantly ran around outside and played sports. Those activities promoted health and body positivity. But as we grew older and hit puberty, the road map for life got a bit crumpled. Raised in a quiet household, we did not talk about controversial or uncomfortable things, and that included our bodies. The things we learned about sex and puberty came directly from awkward, outdated VHS tapes in health class—the kind of movies that were easier to laugh at than pay attention to. Actors with '70s hairstyles and bell-bottoms recited corny dialogue about our changing bodies and what to expect, but no one told us how to adapt to or accept those changes. I wish my parents had told me it was *normal* to gain weight during puberty, and that it was natural as a young woman to have curves and a little bit of fat on my hips. I wish my mom had celebrated my first period in some way—no embarrassing pink confetti or giant tampon-shaped helium balloons necessary—to let me know my body was maturing, and that it was a *good* thing. Instead, she snuck menstrual pads into the deep recesses of the bathroom cabinet, behind the dust bunnies and tile cleaner, never to be mentioned again.

We kept our bodies covered up by wearing shorts and T-shirts over our bathing suits. That behavior stemmed from my mom's deep-rooted insecurities about her own body, and the apple doesn't fall far from the tree. Our bodies became a source of embarrassment and shame. My brother, who was always overweight as a kid, was ashamed when he couldn't perform well in sports like football and skiing, because my dad valued athletic ability over self-esteem. And my weight loss was overlooked because my mom idealized a thin body and dieted herself as a teenager, some days subsisting on a head of iceberg lettuce and Juicy Fruit gum. It took her years to realize that I was *too* thin.

A 2010 study of 356 high school girls found that parental weight-related comments and dieting behaviors, as well as teasing about weight within families, can incite maladaptive behaviors and attitudes toward food in adolescents. Negative body talk has been linked to lower self-esteem, a distorted self-image, and depression, which are in turn risk factors for eating disorders.[7] As little as three to five minutes of weight stigmatization can have a significant impact on body image, according to the *International Journal of Eating Disorders*.[8] And according to a 2023 report in *Nutrients*, the cumulative effect of weight- and diet-related comments, both positive and negative, has been associated with increased psychological distress and body dissatisfaction. In general, while fathers are more likely to tease, mothers are more likely to make comments; when looking at gendered differences, these comments seem to affect the mental well-being of daughters more than sons.[9]

Outside our home, there was little body positivity to be found growing up in the 1990s. The obesity epidemic in the United States began around 1980, with the obesity rate rising from 15.0 percent in the late 1970s to 23.3 percent by the late 1980s.[10] People were dining out more, especially at fast-food restaurants like McDonald's, and the intake of sugar and fat spiked due to the introduction of ultra-processed foods, or UPFs. UPFs are packaged foods that are typically high in calories, sugar, fat, and salt—rich in additives but sometimes completely devoid of nutrition. Many are easy to chew and rapidly consumed, often in portions that exceed the serving size on the label, because they taste so delicious. Packaged cakes, cookies, kids' cereals, and potato chips are good examples of UPFs. They are the same foods that would later play a role in my bulimia. In response to the obesity epidemic, the 1990s introduced fad diets and diet foods, which were ironically just ultra-processed foods with lower calorie counts and cuter names, such as SnackWell's fat-free Devil's Food Cookie Cakes. Everything shifted to "diet" versions—fat-free, sugar-free, low-fat, zero-calorie—in an attempt to make America thin again.

Before the advent of social media, with ads and promotions for every fashion trend and "health hack," we still had traditional media. TV ads and magazines featured waiflike models and promoted diet foods like Special K, a brand that idolized thin women in red bathing suits. "With the help of the K, you can't pinch an inch . . . on me!" the models promised, cinching child-sized belts around their 24-inch waists and eating perfectly measured one-ounce servings of cereal. Amphetamines and "fen-phen," a dangerous combination of the two appetite suppressants fenfluramine and phentermine, hit the market. Diet culture was everywhere, marketed in *Seventeen* and *Cosmopolitan*, magazines that reached a target audience of teenage females, including myself. Instead of showcasing professional female athletes with healthy, muscular bodies, these magazines featured stick-thin models to advertise sports bras and Umbro shorts for young athletes.

Even if you could avoid the media, you couldn't escape age-matched girls comparing themselves in the school bathroom mirrors. Every girl pinched their fat and scrutinized their skin, questioning their self-worth and hoping for a compliment from their friends. *Do I look fat in these pants? Should I skip lunch today? Does this makeup cover my zit? Am I pretty?* In the high school hallways, those feelings of self-doubt were amplified by judgmental stares from other students. Bullying and fat-shaming were done face-to-face before texting and cyberbullying were invented.

I could pinch an inch, maybe more. I was acutely aware of my big thighs and acne without anyone else calling attention to them. But I was still teased. It was impossible not to wish for a thinner body and a prettier face, if only to blend into the crowd and be left alone.

Self-consciousness about our bodies begins as early as elementary school, and it continues to ramp up through puberty and young adulthood. A fifteen-year longitudinal study published in 2020 found that in the US, 24 to 46 percent of adolescent girls and 12 to 26 percent of adolescent boys report marked dissatisfaction with their bodies; this number has increased over time. In general, body dissatisfaction is reported far more often in girls than in boys, and girls who are overweight (BMI 25–29.9) report less body confidence than boys who are clinically obese (BMI >30).[11] Pound for pound, girls are simply less happy in their own skin. It's no wonder I chose a T-shirt and shorts over a hot pink bikini.

Stress

Historically, psychologists and other medical professionals have treated anorexia nervosa as a symptom of an underlying stressor. There "must" have been a trauma or inciting event, some unconscious motive fueling restrictive eating behaviors. Only by addressing the underlying issues could one "fix" their anorexia: Resolve your daddy issues by working on your relationship with your father; find a way to forgive the person who physically or sexually assaulted you; accept the fact that you were dumped; dig deep into your past to see where you lost your self-esteem along the way. This theory was the driver for psychologists to use psychodynamic therapy, a type of talk therapy that can take years—years of chipping away at the underlying problem while the person with anorexia continues to diet and lose weight. Not surprisingly, it comes with high rates of relapse and often a search for other causes.

We now know that anorexia's cause is not so straightforward, and disregarding the nature and nurture that came before the stressor does a disservice to anyone with mental illness. It is impossible to attribute an eating disorder to just *one* factor. In the diathesis-stress model, the stressor is any life event or series of events that disrupts a person's psychological equilibrium. It is the final straw that breaks the camel's back, the last ingredient that makes the pot boil over. It could be anything—the death of a loved one, divorce, physical trauma, social rejection—but that one thing pushes a person across the threshold into mental illness. For me, it was the day my dad's pickup truck drove away down that snowy road.

For too many years, I blamed myself for my eating disorder, for starting a diet that spiraled out of control. I chose to diet, but I never *wanted* to binge or purge, to socially isolate myself, or to make myself unhealthy. At sixteen years old, I was vulnerable, and the eating disorder invaded my body and mind like an opportunistic infection. By the age of thirty, I would be prepared to fight back. I would use the willpower and determination in my prefrontal cortex to extinguish my eating disorder and get healthy again. It would take years to get there, but eventually, I would rewrite my destiny.

Chapter 4

THE ICING ON THE CAKE

Ken and I walked hand in hand across the street as the sun set over the bustling campus quad. We passed by The Cup, our favorite ice cream shop, and despite a desperate urge to eat a huge sundae topped with caramel, whipped cream, and cherries, I kept walking. It was the start of a typical Saturday night at Lehigh University, with underage college students filling Fourth Street in downtown Bethlehem, trying to sneak into any filthy bar that would serve them a beer. We had just finished dinner—thick, greasy slices of four-cheese pizza. For most college students, including my boyfriend, it was a normal "pregaming" meal—something to soak up all the alcohol we would drink later at a Delta Chi frat party. But for me, it was a splurge, a binge. Saturday was a "cheat" day. I was so full, but I wanted to keep eating.

We walked back to the shoddy off-campus townhouse we called home, with its peeling white paint and cheap chain-link fence. Splayed out in bed, hands covering my distended stomach, I tried to will away the fullness before I had to change into a dress. How could I go out and have a good time when I felt so awful, so fat that I was bursting out of my jeans and T-shirt? The bedroom floor was littered with clothes, video games, notebooks, empty soda bottles. Then I spotted a dirty plate and fork sitting on top of the nightstand. It was smeared with thick, oily icing and fluffy crumbs of vanilla cake—the remnants of Funfetti cake, the same cake that had triggered my bulimia.

I knew what I had to do, how to make myself feel better. I told Ken I was going to use the bathroom, to fix my makeup and brush my teeth before we went out. As I left the room, he said, "You're not going to do it, right? Just don't do it. Don't be bad," as if I were a misbehaving child about to write on the walls with crayon. There was some truth in what he said, that simply *not* doing it might help break the destructive habit of bingeing and purging. But in that moment, I lacked the willpower to stop myself. *If he really cares about me, he'll try harder to stop me.* He knew I was bulimic and yet this gentle admonishment was the only thing he did to save me. I closed the bathroom door, leaned over the toilet, and threw up.

———

When I had been accepted to Lehigh University three years earlier, I was ready to escape small-town life and see the world—even if the world was only a bigger town built around old industrial steel stacks an hour west of Blairstown. I was a trailblazer; neither of my parents had attended college. When my mom and I toured the campus, we were awestruck by the layout of stately, historic buildings. Linderman Library, which was over 125 years old, smelled of thousands of worn paperback books and newspapers, and its enormous bay windows invited students to curl up and read while the sunlight streamed in. The Alumni Memorial Building stood as tall and proud as the Statue of

Liberty. Even the dormitories, brick buildings covered in climbing ivy vines, were charming.

We sat in oversized Adirondack chairs on The Quad, watching the steady flow of campus life all around us. It was the only college we toured, and it held the promise of my future. Tuition was $50,000 per year. "Don't worry about the money," my mom said. "We'll figure it out. You can do anything you set your mind to." Nothing was more important than our education; she was hell-bent on raising my sister and me to be smart, independent women. She didn't want us to follow in her footsteps, to rely on a man for financial support. Together, we submitted the Free Application for Federal Student Aid, laughing when it read out "Expected Family Contribution: Zero." Finally, there was validation of how much we had struggled since my dad had left.

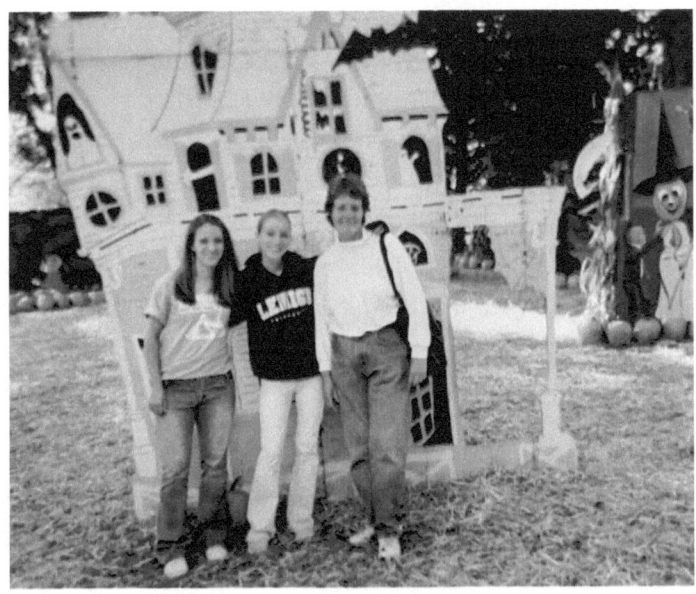

Kerin and my mom and me, circa 2003

Most of my tuition was covered by scholarships and financial aid, but I still needed to work. After class came a work-study job, where I spent hours mindlessly filing papers in manila folders in the financial aid office, followed by evening shifts waiting tables at a mediocre Italian restaurant. Customers who ate bottomless soup and salad for $5.99 would generously toss an entire dollar on the table for my tip, and I salivated over plates of gooey, cheesy baked ziti. The diners didn't know that the lasagna wasn't homemade, that it came from a bulk shipment of frozen Stouffer's, or that I would have given anything for a bite of it.

College was a continuation of bad habits. When I packed my things to move into the dorm, I made sure to bubble-wrap my Wal-Mart scale like fine china, but I forgot to bring my lucky #23 soccer jersey with me. It was too big for me anyway. I was 35 pounds lighter than I had been when I wore it, and at 105 pounds, I still didn't believe I was thin enough. My goal weight, my perfect body, was a moving target, constantly shifting and stretching slightly farther out of reach. I had to try harder. When I wasn't in calculus class, I used my brain to complete rigorous mental calculations of how many calories I ate each day. One granola bar for breakfast (160 calories) + one cup of soup for lunch (125 calories) + one bag of popcorn (150 calories) + salad for dinner (300 calories) = still hungry. Go to sleep and repeat the next day.

But sleep was fitful and unsatisfying. At night I dreamed about all the foods I deprived myself of. In the morning, I woke up feeling achy from the crushing weight of the massive pile of blankets needed to keep me warm and the constant grind of my bony knees on each other while I slept on my side. I knew it wasn't normal to dream about eating a big bowl of cereal and milk. I knew I had an eating disorder; everyone around me knew,

4 | THE ICING ON THE CAKE

but no one dared to say the words out loud. The opposite, in fact: My thinness was applauded by my new friends. Comments like "Wow, I wish I could be as skinny as you" or "I wish I had that kind of self-control" were accepted with a quick smile through gritted teeth. They had no idea I was a starving lunatic, haunted by visions of peanut butter and jelly sandwiches.

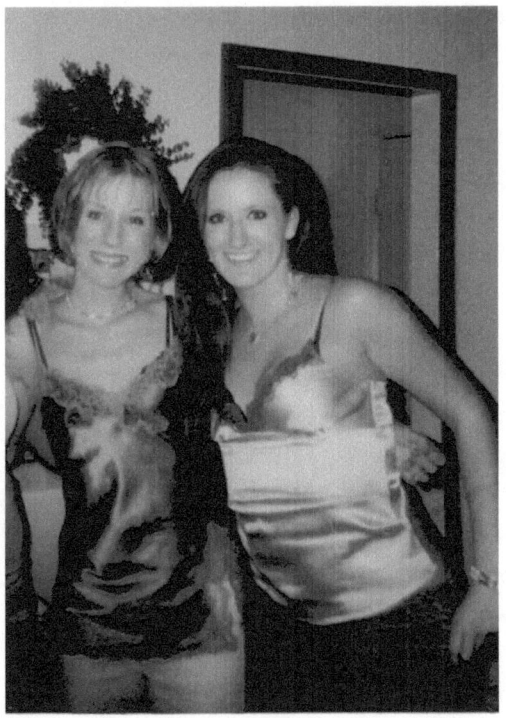

With Kerin, circa 2004

I imagine it pained people to see me eat so little, the same way it had hurt my family when I turned down Thanksgiving dinner and buttery homemade Christmas cookies, so I kept my anorexic behaviors hidden as best I could, eating in the cafeteria at odd hours and pocketing food to eat back in my dorm room by myself. Eating alone meant no suspicious looks about what I had (or didn't have) on my plate, no need for explanations or excuses. On days I treated myself, I indulged in a carefully counted handful of 4-calorie jellybeans after dinner, savoring each one. On days I punished myself, I followed dinner with 100 crunches, trying to burn off the calories I had just eaten. The mini-fridge in my dorm room was stocked with low-fat yogurt, Diet Coke, and Nutri-Grain bars, some of which had been bought by my roommate. She was a beautiful, wealthy sorority pledge-to-be who kept her diet as manicured as her hair and nails. A shared love of diet food seemed to be the only thing we had in common, and she was just as thin as I was. From a thousand freshmen randomly assigned to share dorm rooms, two girls with eating disorders had somehow ended up within the same 250 square feet.

Once a week I dragged myself to the gym to run a mile on the treadmill, convinced that working out was part of a "healthy" routine. Running a mile on a flat treadmill belt felt like running up and down the peaks of the Himalayas. After the first sixty seconds, I was out of breath, forcing myself to lift each foot as effortlessly as if I were wearing lead weights instead of sneakers. I ran in an oversized hoodie and leggings, my shoulders sagging, unable to work up a sweat even though I felt like I was working hard. The athletic clothes I used to own had gotten too big for me and had long ago been discarded as a declaration that I would never have to wear "fat clothes" again. The game-winning goal scorer, the fastest sprinter on the soccer team, was gone, discarded like those clothes. Running, something I had once loved to do, now felt like a chore. I sluggishly jogged until the treadmill hit 1.00 mile, then walked back up the steep hill to my dorm.

"Miss, can you come over here? Did you just put something in your bag?" A cashier in the campus grocery store tried to get my attention as I swept two Yoplait yogurts into my purse. We made eye contact across the room, and I froze in place, trying to figure out my next move. I was standing on a frozen lake, one crack away from falling through thin ice. I could hand over the stolen items and risk being reported, arrested, or worse, kicked out of college, which was the honorable thing to do. Or I could run like hell and hope the ice held my weight.

My obsession with food had reached a dizzying height. I was constantly surrounded by it—in the cafeteria, in the Italian restaurant where I waited tables, at every frat party and social event—but I never allowed myself to eat it. I felt guilty knowing there was a surplus of money on my meal stipend while my mom and sister stared into an empty refrigerator looking for dinner. Most of the kids at Lehigh came from affluent families and were driving Mercedes or BMWs to commute home on the weekend. They emptied their cafeteria trays without a care, oblivious to the fact that they were throwing away nutritious food they had taken but never bothered to touch. They lived in a world of excess and wastefulness, where designer clothes hung unworn in closets and credit card bills were paid by Daddy. I hated them for having it so easy when my family was struggling.

While they threw away their food, I started stockpiling mine, until I had a cache of fresh fruit and snacks to take home to Kerin and my mom on the weekend. Hoarding food quickly turned into stealing food—from the cafeteria, the campus store, even the local supermarket in Bethlehem. I justified it the same way I justified shoplifting clothes: It was a matter of need, not want. Simply *knowing* I had enough food made me feel secure, even if I couldn't eat it. But stealing it only made my relationship with food more twisted. For someone who had worked so hard to get into college, I had no problem risking it all that day for a few yogurts. My heart galloped in my chest as I zipped my bag and darted out of the campus store. Would they call campus security to track me down? I wasn't going to wait around to find out. I ran all the way to my dorm without looking back; fueled by the fear of being caught, I ran faster than I ever had on the treadmill. I would never steal anything again.

When my sister graduated from high school and left for college, I was relieved—one less hungry mouth to feed. She was finally untethered from our childhood home, free to live her life, and her college was only twenty minutes away from mine. I envied Kerin—she was vibrant and fun, a social butterfly who hung out with friends and went to campus parties every weekend. She looked healthy and happy in halter tops, skirts, and flip-flops, a long mane of glossy brown hair flowing down her back. Bright costume jewelry and bold eye makeup, things that might look gaudy on other girls, accentuated her beauty. She wasn't afraid to eat late-night pizza after a bar crawl. Next to her, I felt like a fading star, eclipsed by her brightness. We shared the same emotional scars, but somehow she hid hers like a professional makeup artist while mine were visible to the world. My scars fit into a size 0. When she came to visit me at Lehigh, I let go of my rigid rules and partied like a normal college kid. We had sleepovers and talked into the early hours of the morning, laughing at stupid movies as we tried to throw popcorn into each other's mouths. For just a night, we could forget about our problems and act like sisters again.

I had met Ken halfway through college. He was nerdy, sweet, and easygoing. He was not my first boyfriend, but he was my

4 | THE ICING ON THE CAKE

first love, and his opinion meant everything to me. More like a man twice his age, he had good taste in clothes, cars, and jewelry—he recognized value and beauty. So when he thought I looked beautiful at 100 pounds, with my bony hips jutting out of the top of my jeans and forearms as thin as twigs, I believed him. His admiration validated my anorexia, and that should have been a warning sign. But I was swept away by the maelstrom of young love, where every waking moment revolves around each other and nights are spent touching and talking until the sun comes up. We spent so much time together that it felt natural for me to move into his house junior year. I didn't mind sharing a bed, bathroom, or tube of toothpaste with him, but I wasn't ready to share my secretive, restrictive eating habits.

When we went out to dinner, I ordered a salad with fat-free Italian dressing and a diet soda. "I just like to eat healthy." "I *love* salad." "I don't have a big appetite." I had a grab bag of excuses to explain why I never ate much on our dates, but none of them were true. I loved salads as much as I loved getting a root canal. And my appetite was not the problem. I was starving. I simply wouldn't allow myself to eat. Going out to eat meant being unable to measure my food or study the calorie count of each item on the menu, and that was torture. But he didn't know that.

The longer I stayed with Ken, the safer I felt, and I slowly let my guard down around food. We cheated on my diet "together"; I had an accomplice, and that made me feel less guilty about making bad choices. While I pillaged the fridge, he grabbed utensils and plates, as if I were the robber and he were driving the getaway car. At night, we baked rolls of Pillsbury cookies and ate them in bed while watching movies and playing video games. After sex, we shared a pint of ice cream, chasing one indulgence with another. He didn't seem to mind when I put on a few pounds. "Gain a few more," he encouraged, and I relented.

I thought it would be as simple as flipping a switch, going from a restricted diet to a normal one, adding back all the foods that had been missing, but changing my diet was harder than organic chemistry. Everything I knew about food was wrong, and I didn't know how to make healthy choices anymore. Instead of nutrient-rich foods that would help me build muscle and restore my health, I ate cookies, cake, pizza, and nachos. I was ravenous for all the things I had missed out on for so long.

One afternoon, I was the first to come home from class and decided to bake a cake for Ken. He loved my baking. Baking was a family tradition—Kerin and I had learned to roll cookie dough, pinch pie crusts, and mix cheesecakes as soon as we could recite the alphabet—and it was a way to express love. I pulled out a box of Funfetti cake mix and mixed the batter with eggs and oil before pouring the creamy vanilla cake into round pans. When it was done baking, I smoothed the icing across the golden top and decorated it with rainbow sprinkles. I couldn't wait for him to cut the first piece. Once he did, I could sneak bites of it whenever I wanted, like a mouse slowly nibbling away at it, barely noticeable.

But that day, I wanted the cake so badly that I couldn't resist it. I took a bite out of the corner and put my fork down. Then I picked it back up and took a second bite, then a third, then a fourth. I greedily dug in and ate faster and faster, filling my mouth with sweet vanilla, and suddenly there was no cake left, just crumbs and a smudge of frosting in the pan. I couldn't believe it. How had I eaten an *entire* cake? Where was my self-control? My cheeks flushed with shame. I cleaned up the crime scene, washing the cake pan and hiding the evidence of cracked eggs and scattered crumbs, but the guilt stayed with me. It was a mistake, a one-off; I vowed to never let it happen again.

Weeks later, I ate an entire box of Cinnamon Toast Crunch—

bowl after bowl of sweet, crunchy cereal drowned in milk. Days after that, it was a dozen glazed donuts. Instead of buying a muffin for breakfast on my way to anthropology class, I bought four gigantic cookies—sugar, macadamia nut, chocolate chip, peanut butter—and devoured them, feeling nauseous and ill by the end of class. Every time I binged on unhealthy food, the impulse to binge only got stronger.

Since grocery shopping was done alone, I could pile boxes of Pop-Tarts, Entenmann's donuts, and Chips Ahoy! cookies into my cart without my boyfriend or roommates knowing. Boxes of Little Debbie cakes were $1.09—cheap, devoid of nutrients, and easy to swallow. I hid them around the house, a secret stash of sugar and fat, and ate them when no one was home. Despite my meager budget, my grocery tab grew, as did my desperate need to eat. The grocery store clerks who checked me out time after time probably rolled their eyes to themselves as I carried out enough junk food to feed an army but pleasantly smiled at me anyway and told me to have a nice day.

I could not understand what was causing me to binge eat. Maybe my body was revolting against being too thin. The urge to binge popped up unpredictably and with varying intensity, usually when I was alone, but it didn't seem to matter if I was happy, sad, stressed, or relaxed. Sometimes it would hit me like a tidal wave and pull me under, and I knew I had to binge immediately; afterward, I would resurface, sputtering and splashing, wondering what I had just done. At other times, it would come on gradually like the change of the ocean tide, slowly building within me. I surfed the waves, on some level knowing that the urges were my brain's way of telling me to eat more, to combat the starvation I had forced on myself for so long. But eventually, the urges won, and the waves sent me crashing violently onto the sand.

The DSM-5 criteria for binge eating disorder are as follows:

1. Recurrent episodes of binge eating. An episode of binge eating is characterized by both of the following:
   a. Eating, in a discrete amount of time (e.g., within any two-hour period), an amount of food that is definitely larger than most people would eat in a similar period of time under similar circumstances
   b. The sense of lack of control over eating during the episode (e.g., a feeling that one cannot stop eating or control what or how much one is eating)
2. Binge-eating episodes are associated with three (or more) of the following:
   a. Eating much more rapidly than normal
   b. Eating until feeling uncomfortably full
   c. Eating large amounts of food when not physically hungry
   d. Eating alone because of being embarrassed by how much one is eating
   e. Feeling disgusted with oneself, depressed, or very guilty after overeating
3. Marked distress regarding binge eating is present
4. The binge eating occurs, on average, at least one day a week for three months
5. The binge eating is not associated with the regular use of inappropriate compensatory behavior (e.g., purging, fasting, excessive exercise) and does not occur exclusively during the course of anorexia nervosa or bulimia nervosa.[12]

It was easier to go with the tide than swim against it. I figured gaining weight would quiet the urges that drove me to eat excessively. But the more frequently I acted on the urges, and the more weight I gained, the farther I drifted out to sea. And there was no rescue in sight.

Chapter 5

VANISHING ACT

One hundred twenty-nine pounds. After months of binge eating, I was back to a normal weight. But it didn't look or feel "normal" the way I had hoped it would. It felt uncomfortable and claustrophobic, like a teddy bear overstuffed with polyester filling, ripping at the seams, buttons popping off like bottle tops. The new weight I put on was packed under taut skin and size 0 jeans, with nowhere to go. Stretch marks and cellulite blossomed on my hips and thighs. Overeating junk food left me bloated and nauseous, and my energy level plummeted. I longed to find my "fat clothes" from high school, to dig them out of the Goodwill drop box and relax into their roominess.

The same boyfriend who had encouraged me to eat more no longer wanted to touch me, and I felt like a monster. When he first told me he loved me, I was convinced he would love me no matter what I looked like, but he loved skinny me. And although he would never admit it, he seemed repulsed by my new body—the less attractive, less sexy, heavier version. If he couldn't love me at a normal weight, how was I supposed to love myself? Would I have to starve myself again to feel better?

The summer I spent at the University of Medicine and Dentistry of New Jersey was a respite from the sticky heat and humidity of the East Coast, and a distraction from constantly obsessing about my weight. I was one of a dozen undergraduate students accepted to the neuroscience research program—a group of nerdy, laser-focused college kids who chose academics over beer and sunbathing for eight summer weeks. In the chilly darkness and solitude of the lab, I pored over slides, studying the effects of tumor necrosis factor (TNF)-alpha inhibitors on the oligodendrocytes of mouse brains. My study was only one of many in a massive research lab, and I was an amateur scientist among experts working on therapies for multiple sclerosis.

Looking through the lens of the microscope was much easier than looking in the mirror every day. It was quiet, focused work, the constant whir of the air-conditioning like white noise in the background. While I was working toward a bachelor's degree in biology, I had no idea what I was going to do with the rest of my life. I couldn't imagine spending all my time in a dark lab, isolated from the outside world, unable to see the sun until my lunch break; but I could appreciate the intricate, delicate mesh of neural connections on those tiny glass slides. The dendrites of the neurons lit up in fluorescent greens and blues, creating microscopic tendrils of color. They were beautiful, complex, minuscule works of art. I was fascinated with the idea that we could learn so much from mouse brains. They were smaller and simpler than our human brains, and yet so integral in studying and treating our diseases. It was my first glimpse into the study of neurology.

"We built this program to encourage students to get a PhD and start their own research lab," my mentor told me at the end of the summer. "You should consider getting a PhD or an MD—or both!" Her enthusiasm was contagious. But I couldn't be a bench scientist, sacrificing mice the way the scientists in her lab

5 | VANISHING ACT

did, casually putting pressure on the backs of their necks until they asphyxiated, then dissecting their brains and fixing them on slides. My stomach turned when I watched those mice die.

Maybe I'll be a doctor, I thought. Somehow, in all my years as a straight A student, I had never thought of it. Kids who became doctors were the progeny of doctors, born into wealthy families who could afford medical school, like the premed students at Lehigh University. Kids who became doctors dreamed of being doctors from the time they were five years old, and had Polaroid photos of themselves wearing Fisher-Price stethoscopes and pretending to listen to their moms' hearts. That was never me.

My blue-collar family feared and revered doctors. After my dad left and we no longer had health insurance, we feared the doctor visit's cost as much as the doctor. Trips to the doctor were rare and made only when absolutely necessary. We were expected to take our appointments seriously: We never showed up late, asked too many questions, or challenged the doctor's expertise—and we definitely didn't dress up as doctors on Halloween. No one in my family had ever imagined being a doctor, but I was smart and ambitious—why not go for it? Once the idea entered my mind, I was dead set on it. I was the overachiever, and I would continue to overachieve. My single-minded focus was just one example of the all-or-nothing, black-or-white, rigid way of thinking that had gotten me into trouble when I started dieting, but this decision felt like a better use of it. I started studying for the Medical College Admission Test (MCAT) right away.

Despite my newfound purpose, the eating disorder was lying in wait, ready to pounce as soon as I returned to campus for senior year. Ken and I sat at a table in the campus quad, where I buried my nose in MCAT prep materials and sipped on unsweetened iced tea. I still had no idea how to eat normally. I alternated between days of fasting and days of bingeing like an animal darting back and forth in the headlights of a car unsure of which way to go, and this was another day of restriction. "You haven't eaten much today. Have some of these," he offered gently, pushing a big bag of potato chips across the table.

The gesture was done with good intention, but he could no longer predict my reaction, as I was constantly conflicted about food. One moment I thanked him for being sweet; the next I snapped at him for pressuring me to eat. One day I starved; the next I feasted. *Don't feed me fucking chips when I'm already getting fat*, I thought angrily. Swallowing my feelings instead of those salty, crunchy chips, I pushed the bag back across the table with a silent shake of my head. I simultaneously loved him and hated him, the same way I loved and hated food. But it wasn't his fault. He was trying to help me the only way he knew how, by giving me something to eat when I was hungry. I needed *real* help.

Since starting to binge eat, I felt embarrassed and ashamed of my eating habits and weight gain. I missed being anorexic. I *liked* being regimented and in control of my diet, and now I felt directionless and anxious. There was something wrong with me, some reason I could not control myself around food. That realization led me to the front door of the university's mental health resources building. As a student, a soft knock and a cry for help were all I needed to gain free access to a psychologist. It seemed too good to be true when the rest of the world had to pay hundreds of dollars out of pocket.

But the first attempt with individual therapy was short-lived. The therapist sat calmly with her legs crossed, her face unreadable, and spoke in hushed tones as she asked me how I felt in a way that made me want to cry. She asked about my home life, my parents, symptoms of depression, self-harm, suicidal thoughts. I wasn't suicidal; I just wanted someone to tell me how to stop stuffing my damn face with junk food. Tears bubbled up, and I bit them back, refusing to cry. I hated crying, especially in front of complete strangers. Talking to a therapist was supposed to be *easier* than talking to someone close to me—a place to reveal my inner thoughts without fear of judgment—but I was affronted by it. Her questions felt intrusive and probing. Like a turtle retreating into its shell, I withdrew and never showed up for the next appointment.

Group therapy was better, at first. There were strategies, the therapist told us, to distract the mind from fixating on food and using maladaptive eating behaviors. We were told to make lists of activities, hobbies, and meditations we could use as substitutes for obsessing over food. They were good tools to use, if we could actually put them into practice once we left the therapy room. Art was one of the many suggested distractions, and our therapist also taught the basics of acrylic painting. So instead of coffee and pastries at the group sessions, we were given blank canvases. The room reminded me of a kindergarten classroom, with stackable plastic chairs placed in a semicircle and bins of art supplies off to the side.

I was skeptical that art could be a cure for my problems, but I was willing to give it a try. "Run your brush across the canvas in long sweeping strokes, then mix a bit of purple in to create a darker hue," the therapist instructed. We painted the sunset over the beach, blending streaks of pink, orange, and purple across the sky—calming imagery for turbulent minds. But outside the room, would I be able to reach for a paintbrush before reaching into the box of glazed Pop'ems? It seemed easier said than done, but I felt some progress.

The therapist asked us to share our thoughts around the

circle—even those of us who were usually quiet. Every time I spoke, my heart jumped into my throat and my fear of public speaking tightened its grip. The easel in front of me was a shield, its frame a thin wall of protection from complete vulnerability. When I was done sharing, I turned back to my painting, sweeping the brush across the canvas until my anxiety dissipated and my grip on the paintbrush loosened. But the more I talked, the more comfortable I felt. The other girls echoed my thoughts—they understood me, and I no longer felt alone. It was a safe space for the sisterhood hidden within Lehigh's student body.

Everything was going well until the day Cathy appeared. We exchanged a quick wave and smile across the circle, then glanced down, momentarily embarrassed that we had run into each other in therapy instead of chemistry class. She was skinny, but I had no idea she was anorexic. Somehow I had become so preoccupied with my own illness that I could no longer recognize it in others. It seemed like every time I attended, another familiar face appeared. There was the thin soccer player who had put on weight quickly and then disappeared from the team, the girl with piercings who worked in the campus bookstore, another classmate I had partnered with in calculus. There were too many girls who recognized me, and I wasn't sure they could keep my secret. It suddenly felt like my problems were on display for the entire student body, one step away from a gigantic highway billboard sign of my face towering over the campus. "Come see the disappearing girl!" it would advertise. "Now you see her; now you don't!" I felt as exposed as a circus performer under a harsh spotlight, all eyes on me. I wanted help but only if it came with complete anonymity. The only option was to leave the stage and go back into the darkness, to quit group and find another way to get better.

Therapy takes time, and I was impatient. I ran away from

group therapy without looking at the path ahead of me, and ran right into a bigger problem. One terrible evening changed the course of my illness irrevocably. It was a long day at work, and my feet ached from running laps around the restaurant, serving plate after plate of chicken parmesan for ten hours straight. The smell of marinara sauce clung to my clothes and lingered in my nostrils. Exhausted, I sat down at the table with a carry-out container of baked ziti, a kickback for my hard work, and the rolled-up cash I made in tips. I was $150 richer, and my stomach was growling. But as soon as I finished eating, I felt uncomfortably full, gluttonous, disgusting.

I couldn't take it anymore. I had to get rid of the food that was weighing me down like an anchor. *Just make yourself throw up*, the voice in my head said. *You'll feel so much better.* Hesitantly, I walked to the bathroom, knelt on the cold, hard tiles next to the toilet, and stuck my finger in the back of my throat. I felt a rising sensation and a buildup of pressure behind my eyes as I got rid of everything I had just eaten. When I opened my eyes again, my face was flushed and my eyes were bloodshot from the effort. I gasped for air. First, there was horror at what I had done, but then came a rush of relief. The anxiety was gone. No one had witnessed what I had done, and much like my first binge, I could pretend my first purge had never happened.

Like bingeing, I thought I would do it only once. Every time thereafter, I told myself the same lie: *This is the last time. Tomorrow is your chance to start over.* I reset the clock daily, weekly, monthly. But the need to repeat the behavior overtook all rational thought, and I always eventually gave in. No longer would friends or family comment on how little I was eating or cast judgmental glances at my plate, because now I could eat a normal meal in their eyes. They didn't need to know what happened after.

It was a high-stakes magic trick, making food disappear.

Instead of smoke and mirrors, I hid behind a bathroom door. The prestige, the grand finale, was that I still looked like a normal college student when I reappeared. The behavior was invisible to anyone else. The more I did it, the more seamless it became. It was alarming how quickly a revolting behavior could become part of my daily routine. When I told my boyfriend and he brushed it off as nothing more than a bad habit, so did I.

In my attempt to run away from anorexia, I had jumped a hurdle into bulimia. Bulimia was the secretive, less obvious eating disorder that hid behind a normal weight. While it is fairly common to go from anorexic to bulimic, I didn't know that then, and I didn't know how or why it happened to me.

According to the DSM-5, bulimia nervosa is defined as:

1. Recurrent episodes of binge eating, as characterized by both:
   a. Eating, within any 2-hour period, an amount of food that is definitively larger than what most individuals would eat in a similar period of time under similar circumstances.
   b. A feeling that one cannot stop eating or control what or how much one is eating.
2. Recurrent inappropriate compensatory behaviors in order to prevent weight gain, such as self-induced vomiting; misuse of laxatives, diuretics, or other medications; fasting or excessive exercise.
3. The binge eating and inappropriate compensatory behaviors occur, on average, at least once a week for 3 months.
4. Self-evaluation is unjustifiably influenced by body shape and weight.
5. The disturbance does not occur exclusively during episodes of anorexia nervosa.[13]

5 | VANISHING ACT

I was determined to move forward with my life, even if I had to juggle mental health issues and bad habits. My next act would be a tightrope walk, balancing an eating disorder with becoming a doctor.

Chapter 6

THE CHEMISTRY OF CONTENTMENT

Think of the brain as a house. The rooms downstairs, such as the laundry room and the kitchen, perform basic functions. These are the primitive areas of the brain, responsible for breathing, blinking, fight-or-flight responses, and other reflexive functions that keep us alive. The ensuite bathroom and walk-in closet are upstairs. These are the more sophisticated, evolved parts of our brain, such as the prefrontal cortex. But the layout of the house is almost beside the point. What keeps it running is the electricity, the plumbing, and constant communication between family members. My job as a vascular neurologist, taking care of stroke patients, is not so different from that of a plumber; I just use clot-busting medications instead of Drano to clear out the pipes—that is, the clogged arteries.

In the brain, neurons communicate by electrical and chemical signals. The chemical messengers are called neurotransmitters, and they create the constant chatter between cells. Neurons need to communicate as effectively as people living under the same roof. Talking too much or too little or angrily shouting up the stairs can disrupt the household as much as a power outage can.

Sometimes the dishwasher overflows, a hair dryer trips the circuit breaker, or a lightbulb goes out. In people with eating disorders, the problems at home are not limited to one area. We have over- and underactive parts of our brains as well as structural differences that fluctuate with the state of our illness, from acutely sick to chronically sick to recovered. And we definitely have problems with communication. Our brains are different from those of people without eating disorders, and we know this thanks to new brain imaging techniques such as functional magnetic resonance imaging (usually known as functional MRI or fMRI) and fluorodeoxyglucose–positron emission tomography scans (usually shortened to FDG-PET scans). A review of all the brain changes found in people with eating disorders is beyond the scope of this book (it belongs in a 700-page hardcover book in a medical school library, collecting dust with the other tomes).

Instead, I'll focus on two important neurotransmitters implicated not only in eating disorders but also in mood disorders and schizophrenia: serotonin and dopamine.

Serotonin

Our brains, like our bodies, seek equilibrium. To maintain homeostasis, the brain needs a consistent balance of neurotransmitters, the most common ones being the monoamines (for the chemistry nerds, these are molecules that have an amino group connected to an aromatic ring by a two-carbon chain), which includes serotonin, dopamine, epinephrine (adrenalin), and norepinephrine. Neurons communicate like family members, sending these chemical messages back and forth. When a parent announces that dinner is ready, the kids come running—receiving the message

6 | THE CHEMISTRY OF CONTENTMENT

with both their ears and their hungry stomachs. With neurons, the message is received by specific cell receptors, which are proteins typically found on the surface of cells. Different shape proteins accept different types of messages; they must "fit" like a lock and key. When a receptor receives a chemical message, it internalizes it—that is, sends it into the cell. Cells are packed closely together, with the space between them so small—only 20 to 40 nanometers wide—that it is invisible to the human eye. (By comparison, a human hair is about 80,000 to 100,000 nanometers wide.) That space is called a synapse, and messages travel across synapses at breakneck speed.

Serotonin, a chemical secreted by the brain and gut, is intrinsically involved in mood, sleep, memory, and appetite. Low serotonin levels lead to poor mood, anxiety and depression, aggression, and even suicidal tendencies. New research suggests that low serotonin may even be implicated in long COVID symptoms such as fatigue and "brain fog."

Serotonin levels are partly dependent on our diet, since serotonin is made from tryptophan, an essential amino acid ("essential" meaning it can't be made by our bodies). Tryptophan is found in many animal-based foods (meat, poultry, dairy) but also in many grains, nuts and seeds, and some vegetables; it is the same amino acid that gets blamed when you fall asleep after eating turkey at Thanksgiving. Even modest dieting can decrease the availability of tryptophan and therefore serotonin in the brain. Low serotonin levels can be an indicator of starvation or, in the case of a troubled teenager, a diet that goes too far.

You've heard the phrase "you are what you eat." But with serotonin, it's more like "you are what you are *before* you eat." There are genetic differences that affect the way our brains use and process serotonin, which means that some people are more prone to imbalances in serotonin levels than others. For instance, there are differences based on sex; females tend to have more dramatic responses to changes in serotonin than males, which is one reason females may be more likely to develop eating disorders. Additionally, in people who recover from an eating disorder, some of the disorder-related changes we see in the brain persist, suggesting that the differences may be innate to that individual's brain chemistry—a *cause* rather than an effect of an eating disorder.

When serotonin levels drop far enough, the brain tries to compensate by increasing the number of cell receptors that collect serotonin. Imagine that you are waiting for rain in the middle of a drought. You can put out one bucket to collect the rain when it falls; that might get you a few drops of water to quench your thirst. Or you can put out a hundred buckets, so that when it rains you collect enough water to cook with or fill a bathtub. The brain puts out a hundred buckets.

While anorexia and bulimia are behaviorally opposed—restricting versus bingeing—serotonin is serotonin, and low levels of it cause similar symptoms, but with variable severity. When the brain puts out extra buckets to catch serotonin, ideally a steady rain will fill the buckets gradually and resolve the drought. But for a patient with anorexia, the long-awaited rain—in this case eating or bingeing after being starved—feels like a torrential downpour, saturating the ground and flooding the buckets so fast that they topple over. When a patient with anorexia starts eating again—or worse, bingeing—serotonin levels surge and overwhelm the brain, creating a feeling of anxiety and emotional lability. I experienced this surge of emotions the first time I ate an entire Funfetti cake, and it was not pleasant. And for patients with bulimia, a period of fasting creates an even more drastic decline in serotonin levels, which leads to stronger symptoms, compensatory bingeing, and correspondingly stronger serotonin surges. If someone with anorexia experiences a rainstorm, someone with bulimia experiences a hurricane. While binge eating disorder is less studied than anorexia and bulimia, it seems to follow similar trends as bulimia, with carbohydrate binges triggering similar responses in the brain.

Dopamine

Dopamine, often called the "pleasure" chemical, is the brain's most important neurotransmitter for reward processing. It is released when we are pursuing a reward or *anticipating* a reward, and it makes us seek out and crave that reward again, even if the reward is maladaptive. Things that can get you in trouble—illicit drug use, gambling, sex addiction—are all ways to get a dopamine hit, but getting arrested, going bankrupt, and overdosing are not pleasurable outcomes. The fun is in the chase.

Dopamine plays a big role in binge eating, bulimia, and other obsessive-compulsive behaviors. That is because food is a potent activator of the reward system in the brain, an area called the nucleus accumbens. We love food: It can trigger the reward pathways when we are hungry, when we are actively thinking about our next meal, when we smell food, and even during the actual process of eating. The biggest triggers are calorically dense, highly palatable foods like pizza and cake—the things most likely to be consumed on a "binge day."

As with serotonin, and reemphasizing the importance of nature versus nurture, there are inherent factors (genetic changes that impact dopamine signaling) and conditional ones (such as dieting or restricting food) that can affect levels of dopamine in the brain and make a person more likely to develop an eating disorder. Periods of "hedonic deprivation," where palatable foods are restricted or not consumed, can make the brain feel more needy and us more likely to indulge in compensatory overeating once food becomes available. This is the pattern I later fell into during medical residency, when I had several days of fasting or "clean" eating, only to be followed by intense bingeing episodes. Purging, while not a pleasurable remedy, was the price to pay for my brain seeking a food-induced dopamine fix. People with anorexia and bulimia have been found to have altered neurologic responses to food-related stimuli, in terms of both dopamine levels and an emotional dysregulation that comes with eating. Loss of control, despair, and hopelessness are some of the most commonly reported symptoms of binge eaters. Binge eating does not feel good, but the craving for food and the desire to binge is irresistible.

While dopamine may be notorious for the negative behavior patterns it can trigger, it is not in and of itself "bad"; it is a chemical necessary for survival. It plays a role in heart rate and blood pressure regulation, kidney function, digestion, memory and learning, and motor movements. Ask anyone with Parkinson's disease: I'm sure they'd prefer to have *more* dopamine. In Parkinson's disease, dopaminergic neurons degenerate in a part of the brain called the substantia nigra, and lack of dopamine leads to tremors, balance issues, rigidity, and trouble initiating movements; walking becomes difficult, limited by shuffling steps and frequent falls, and it only gets worse over time. Dopamine also drives goal-directed behaviors necessary for life, including eating—not bingeing, just regular eating. Studies show that genetically engineered dopamine-depleted mice lose their initiative to move and eat; without dopamine, they eventually die. The same fate would hold true for humans.

The Minnesota Starvation Experiment, now considered

somewhat unethical, showed what can happen when we mess with serotonin and dopamine levels.[14] Conducted near the end of World War II to look at the effects of starvation and strategies for effective dietary rehabilitation (re-feeding), and intended to guide the Allies' postwar relief efforts, the experiment enrolled a group of healthy men who were conscientious objectors and volunteered for the study as an alternative to enlisting. When their calories were severely restricted for twenty-four weeks, they lost weight and their metabolism slowed, as might be expected, but the most profound effects were on their mood and thinking.

The men became depressed, moody, socially withdrawn, and preoccupied with food, collecting recipes, performing odd rituals with their food, and chewing gum excessively. They had no interest in sex or physical activity, only food. Effects on mood and thinking were even worse during recovery, when they were allowed to eat unrestricted amounts of food. They didn't know how to go back to eating normally. Many of the men binged, some stole food and ate out of trash cans, and their appetites seemed to be ravenous and insatiable; they gained weight, often exceeding the weight at which they started. The men became anxious, irritable, and impulsive. Some needed years of therapy to cope to return to normal eating. This study shed light on the neurobiology of eating disorders, and it explains why I could not "cure" my anorexia by eating normally: My brain would not allow it.

As it turns out, our brains hate being deprived or starved in any way. Deprivation due to poverty, food insecurity, and other socioeconomic disparities can make a person more likely to seek things that give them instant gratification and a quick dopamine high—things like drugs and alcohol. A 2018 study in *Addiction & Health* found that people with an annual income below

$20,000 were 36 percent more likely to have substance abuse problems than those with an income above $75,000; and unemployed people were twice as likely as full-time workers to struggle with addiction.[15] The people with the least money to spend are the ones most likely to develop gambling, shopping, and nicotine addictions that put them further in debt. When my family was poor, we contributed to these statistics; my mom turned to alcohol and cigarettes while I became a kleptomaniac and a binge eater.

Related Illnesses

Because serotonin and dopamine are so intimately involved in mood and behavior, there is a significant overlap between eating disorders, mood disorders, and anxiety disorders. Mood disorders have a much higher lifetime prevalence in people with eating disorders compared to the general population, occurring in up to 42 percent, 46 percent, and 70 percent of individuals with anorexia, binge eating disorder, and bulimia, respectively.[16]

According to the Anxiety and Depression Association of America, two-thirds of people with an eating disorder will experience an anxiety disorder at some point in their life.[17] The most common co-occurrence is obsessive-compulsive disorder, or OCD, which is characterized by recurrent thoughts and impulses that cause distress or anxiety (obsessions) and compensatory repetitive behaviors to reduce stress and respond to those impulses (compulsions). Replace "obsession" with "the urge to binge eat" and "compulsion" with "binge and purge" and you have bulimia. All these conditions are intertwined.

During my illness, I gave in to many obsessive and compulsive behaviors. Bingeing and purging was by far the worst. I also chewed gum excessively like the men in the starvation study, burning through packs of sugar-free gum like a chain-smoker with a carton of Marlboros. And I chewed food and spit it out instead of swallowing; I thought this trick to avoid overeating was something I had cleverly made up, but it is actually a well-known compulsive behavior called rumination that is common to people with eating disorders. Cooking shows and recipe books were like porn for my anorexic brain.

In residency, binge drinking and partying were how I let loose and relaxed after a long workweek. I did not realize that those behaviors, while normal for many twenty-somethings living in a city, were also entangled with my bulimia. Many people with eating disorders struggle with substance use, especially binge drinking. Binge drinking is a short, intense episode of overconsumption to the point of intoxication, with an associated feeling of loss of control. It is often defined as consuming enough alcohol to raise the blood alcohol concentration (BAC) to 0.08% or higher; this corresponds to consuming four or more drinks for women, or five or more drinks for men, within a two-hour period. Binge drinking is the cousin of binge eating, except that it is more socially acceptable. When you knock back shots at the bar to the point of falling over, you're the life of the party; when you binge eat an entire box of cookies and a gallon of ice cream while playing giant Jenga, you're a social outcast. It's time to go home. Binge eating is secretive and better done alone.

Binge drinking activates the same reward pathways in the brain, and can also stimulate intense hunger, which is why many people raid the fridge or eat a late-night meal after drinking. A slice of pizza at 2 a.m. might be okay for the average person. But for someone with an eating disorder, binge drinking leads to disinhibition and potentiates binge eating behaviors. For me, drinking galvanized my desire to engage in impulsive behaviors—

not just bingeing but also excessive spending at the bar, staying up until all hours of the night, and one-night stands. When I drank too much, I risked my safety walking home alone on unsafe streets and through dark alleyways. Once the first tequila shot was taken, all the dominoes fell . . .

Finding Equilibrium

Chemical changes in the brain are the basis for the pharmacologic treatment of mood disorders and eating disorders. The phrases "happy pills" and "Prozac nation" come to mind when we think of antidepressants, a class of medication used to treat both conditions. Antidepressants are everywhere, as ubiquitous as Motrin and Benadryl. The most commonly used are selective serotonin reuptake inhibitors, a.k.a. SSRIs, which increase the amount of serotonin available in synapses. There are also antidepressants called norepinephrine and dopamine reuptake inhibitors (NDRIs) that increase the amount of dopamine available; Wellbutrin, which is also used to stop smoking, is a good example.

It would be great if a single pill could prevent the bucket from running dry or spilling over. Unfortunately, it is not that simple. Medications often come with side effects—weight gain, headaches, nausea, sexual dysfunction, suicidal thoughts—that can be less tolerable than the symptoms of the illness itself. For Parkinson's patients, medications that augment dopamine can lead to impulse control disorders, such as pathologic gambling, and uncontrollable movements of their arms and legs known as dyskinesias. Modern medicine can't fix everything.

The DSM-5 mentions nothing of these chemical imbalances when it comes to the definition or treatment of eating disorders. Most psychiatric illnesses are diagnosed based on reported symptoms, rather than on lab tests or neuroimaging. If you have hallucinations and delusions, you might have schizophrenia. If you have recurrent intrusive thoughts and urges, you might have OCD. "Intense fear of gaining weight or becoming fat, despite being underweight" is a subjective symptom of anorexia, unmeasurable by anyone other than the person experiencing it. Therefore, the effectiveness of treatment for eating disorders is judged based on improvement of self-reported symptoms; improved mood and a healthier relationship with food are the intangible results patients strive for. Gaining weight or reaching a target "healthy" weight is by no means curative.

The treatment of eating disorders is still heavily reliant on psychotherapy to address maladaptive behaviors and perceptions related to self-image and food. The key to seeking treatment is first recognizing that there *is* a problem. Many people with anorexia are on a crusade for perfection and often view therapy as unnecessary or counterproductive. Being thin is the goal, and the drive to achieve that goal is ego-syntonic, meaning that the goal aligns with that person's ego, or true sense of self. Anorexia gave me purpose and a sense of control, and that made my ego happy. It was only when I started binge eating that I realized I needed help. Bingeing brought unwelcome weight gain and uncomfortable symptoms like bloating and nausea. My face was puffy, and my eyes were bloodshot from vomiting. I felt as awful as I looked, and the urges in my brain telling me to binge and purge were ego-dystonic—that is, no longer in agreement with who I was at the core.

Cognitive behavioral therapy (CBT), which focuses on thoughts, behaviors, and feelings toward eating and works to change attitudes toward weight and body image, is one of the most effective therapies for people with eating disorders, but there are plenty of other options. Psychodynamic psychotherapy, as I mentioned earlier, focuses on addressing any underlying stressors or unconscious conflicts that affect one's relationship with body image and food. For me, that would be resolving my "daddy issues" related to abandonment. Biofeedback is another technique that teaches awareness of the effects of stress on your physiology, including changes in heart rate, breathing, skin temperature, and muscle tension, so that you can better control the body's reaction to stress. As part of the recovery process, family-based therapies engage relatives and loved ones to encourage healthy eating, promote a normal weight, and discourage negative behaviors.

Sadly, only one in ten people with an eating disorder seeks help. And of those who do, many will relapse despite treatment with medication and psychotherapy. According to a 2018 systematic review of studies looking at anorexia nervosa specifically, the rate of relapse was 31 percent, and the risk of relapse was highest in the first year; these statistics held true across all age groups.[18] A 2022 paper that included nineteen studies looking at outcomes and risk of relapse in people with anorexia found the relapse rate at twelve months to be even higher, at 50 percent. These studies found that predictors of relapse at the end of treatment included BMI below or near the lower end of normal—that is, not putting on "enough" weight—as well as duration of illness, severity, and bingeing-purging behaviors associated with anorexia.[19] Additionally, the relapse risk is higher for those with anorexia than for those with bulimia or binge eating disorder. In the end, fewer than half of those with an eating disorder will achieve full remission or recovery.

If it all comes down to a flip of the coin, was I just one of the lucky ones? As an undergrad, I briefly tried individual therapy but didn't feel comfortable with my therapist. I tried group cognitive behavioral therapy, but it felt like an unwanted breach

6 | THE CHEMISTRY OF CONTENTMENT

of privacy. Maybe I didn't try hard enough, or maybe these approaches simply weren't the right fit. Hospitalization was too costly to consider. I never tried antidepressants, but there were plenty of times I felt depressed or anxious enough to warrant one.

I've learned that the road to recovery is not a straight line. And even though our brains share the same chemical pathways, we can each choose our own unique recovery path. The key is finding equilibrium, and I found less conventional ways to achieve it, as you will see. I restored the cocktail of mood-stabilizing chemicals in my brain without a pill. Eventually, I discovered two powerful remedies that were stronger than anything Western medicine could offer me, and they were the things that would ultimately heal me from my eating disorder: endurance sports and nature.

Chapter 7

MAKING THE CUT

A horde of eager students gathered around the professor in the anatomy lab. It was my first day of medical school, and I peered over the shoulders of my new classmates to get a glimpse of the long metal tray table. On it lay an exposed cadaver, one of twelve spaced evenly around the room. "Five students to a body," the prof said casually, as if we were being divided into kickball teams. We dispersed, and he gave us an overview of the course and taught us about the dissection tools we would be using. He asked for a moment of silence to honor the people whose bodies had been graciously donated to our medical education, and he introduced some of them by name, occupation, and age. That was when reality set in: I was about to dissect a human body.

I stood with my gloved hands clasped in front of my scrubs, trembling at the idea of having to cut into the preserved skin and muscle in front of me. The smell of formaldehyde made me dizzy; I would never get used to the odor. *I can't believe I'm here.* Then I remembered all the reasons I wanted to be there: I was there to put my ambition and drive toward something meaningful; to make my family proud; to stretch the limits of my ability to learn and use knowledge; to help people. Being there was a chance to be brave. Selfishly, I wondered if med school would distract my mind enough to liberate me from the bad behaviors that had followed me from college. *Medical school and residency will be hard,* I thought. *Surely I'll have to give up the eating disorder if I want to be successful as a doctor.* There was no turning back; I picked up the scalpel and made the first cut.

Med school redefined for me the concepts of studying and working hard. For the first time in my life, I questioned if I was a good student. I could no longer study for an hour, pass an exam, and then forget the material as I had done so many times in high school and college. When I failed my first biochemistry exam, the bold red F on the paper stung like a slap in the face. I was shocked: I had never failed any test in my life. The material I learned in medical school would need to be incorporated into every fiber of my being, etched into memory to be recalled at any moment in the future when I needed it. When I became a doctor, patients, families, and nurses would expect me to think on my feet; in an emergency, there would be no time to pull out a textbook.

When it came to my college GPA and MCAT score, I hit all the marks, but I was surprised that a strong academic performance was the only requirement to get into medical school, especially since physicians top the list of professions with the highest suicide rates. Didn't anyone want to know if my mental health was intact before I jumped into four years of intense schooling followed by three to six years of residency boot camp? Adopting a dog from a shelter required more rigorous psychological

7 | MAKING THE CUT

screening: *Will you have enough time and love to give to your pet? Can you handle the stress of a pet on top of your work schedule? Will you be a* good *pet owner?* There was no mental health screening to get into medical school, but there should have been—and I would have failed it just like I failed my biochemistry test. Instead, I was welcomed into Robert Wood Johnson Medical School in the summer of 2007. Failing my first exam was a wake-up call that I needed to try harder.

What were the attributes of a good med school student? When it came to raw intelligence, it was an even playing field. Chances were high that the person next to you in physiology was also once a valedictorian or salutatorian, an honors student, a member of the "gifted and talented" group in school. The only way to distinguish yourself was to study harder than everyone else, and that meant spending all your waking hours in the study hall or library. My classmates set the bar high with their dedication, bringing frozen dinners and toothbrushes with them to school every day so that they could spend the evening hours there studying. It was a competition to see who could study the longest, and the last car in the parking lot proclaimed the winner. The ones who spent the most time away from their homes, who sacrificed relationships and sleep, were called "gunners." The gunners were workaholics, addicted to studying like I was addicted to food. While I was willing to up my studying game, I was not ready to relinquish all of my freedom.

"Do you want veggie lo mein or fried rice tonight?" my roommate asked. Erin and I had made a pact to never eat dinner in the school library. Instead, we ate on our drab, olive-green couch, laughing at episodes of *Jersey Shore* on MTV with Chinese takeout containers and pharmacology handouts sprawled across the coffee table. Our two-bedroom garden apartment was a sanctuary at the end of a long day of classes.

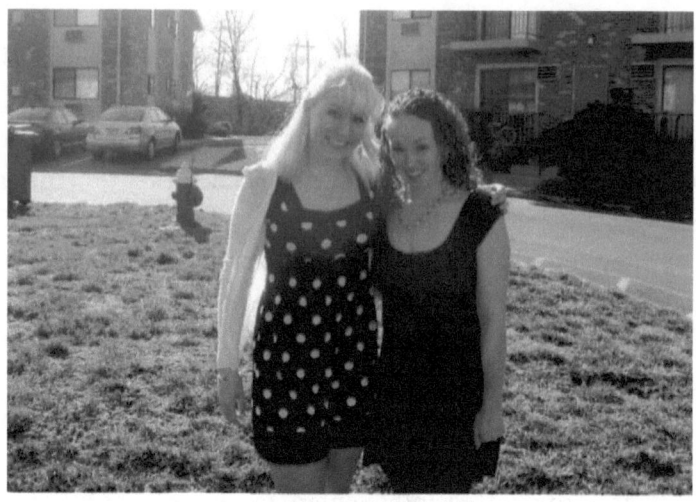

With my med school roommate, Erin

Like me, Erin came from a working-class family and knew the value of hard work, but she also knew how to unwind. She took care of herself, ate a balanced diet, and exercised as part of her daily routine, and she looked healthy because of it. Her freckled face was pretty without any makeup, and she was comfortable in her own skin. For someone in her twenties, she had her shit together.

Instead of following the gunners at school, I followed Erin like I was her little sister. She was the first healthy female role model I had met since playing soccer. After class, she showed me how to use the elliptical and the weight machines at the campus gym. We worked out side by side, propping up microbiology handouts on the elliptical, reading the bouncing text as we worked our arms and legs.

We started preparing lunches and dinners together, and I began eating much cleaner, more nutritious foods from day to day because of it. When she cooked, it was easy for her to portion food without overdoing it—one piece of chicken, a side of rice, steamed veggies—so I copied her. I followed her around the grocery store, throwing into my cart the same items she picked off the shelves. Bingeing and purging ebbed as I learned to feel satisfied with eating a real meal instead of snacking or overeating junk food. During lunch, I studied with my friends, and instead of staring lustfully at their sandwiches, I pulled out my own brown bag holding a bagel, an apple, and pretzels. I felt proud of myself for packing lunch. I was being normal, and normal felt good.

When spring arrived, we were restless from too much time spent studying indoors, from watching the cold, gray blanket of winter through our apartment windows. "Let's go for a run at Johnson Park," Erin suggested. I was nervous to start running again; I hadn't done it since high school soccer. My pathetic attempts to run a mile on the treadmill at Lehigh stuck in my mind, a reminder that I was *not* a runner and I probably never would be. Toward the end of college, I had binged so much that I hit an uncomfortable 165 pounds. With every step and bounce of the elliptical machine, I could feel the extra weight on my hips and stomach rubbing against the fabric of my cotton T-shirt. The elliptical workouts helped me shed a few pounds and feel better, but I wasn't sure if I would be able to run. Running was hard, and I was starting back at zero.

The loop was four miles along flat pavement, weaving through a playground and picnic area and passing in front of the Rutgers football stadium, where red flags marking the entrance flapped gently in the breeze. "We'll just take it easy and see how far we get," Erin said. I nodded. When we finished the first mile, I was as proud as if I had run a marathon. By the end of the second mile, I was panting and huffing, sweating through the cheap Hanes undershirt I had bought at Wal-Mart to exercise in. We took a break to walk.

Salty beads of sweat dampened my bangs and dripped down the side of my face. My thighs rubbed together, chafing from the friction. Without a watch to keep pace, time was marked only by the sound of our steps, and it seemed to stretch on and on. It was effortful, but at the end of the loop, I felt accomplished. We ran only four miles, but that was the farthest I had ever run. And it was the first time in years that exercising felt right, like I was doing something good for my body. My muscles remembered the act of running, and they liked it.

From that day on, every Saturday morning was spent at Johnson Park. We slept in, had breakfast, and then hit the pavement. We filled our noses and lungs with fresh air, a welcome break from the smell of anatomy lab. Running was freeing, and it was free. It didn't require any expensive gear, just shorts, beat-up old sneakers, and a fifteen-dollar six-pack of undershirts. It was the perfect sport for two girls who didn't have a lot of money.

When my roommate was busy, I went by myself, jogging slowly along the path, pop music blaring from the iPod mini clipped to my shorts. My running form and speed were terrible, but I didn't let that crush me. I had once been an athlete, and she was still in there somewhere. Maybe if I kept running, I would find her. I started running more and more on my own, along the sidewalks in my neighborhood and on the treadmill at the gym. Before I knew it, I was running five to six miles at a time.

I was finally hitting my stride, on the pavement and in school. I never failed a test again; in fact, I worked my way up to the top 20 percent of the class and was chosen for the Alpha Omega Alpha Honor Medical Society. Things were going great.

But bulimia was still the monster lurking in the shadows, ready to reach out and grab me when I was vulnerable. When I felt stressed before an exam, when I fought with my boyfriend, when I spent a weekend at home and saw my mom burying her depression beneath a pile of cigarette butts, when I was left alone with my thoughts at night, unable to fall asleep, it was there.

Bingeing was a coping mechanism for stress, a shoulder to cry on, a comfort when things felt out of control. Like a chain-smoker cutting down to half a pack per day, I had curbed the bingeing and purging behaviors, but they weren't gone. They still consumed my daily thoughts. Sometimes I bargained with myself: *No bingeing or purging for one week.* Then, *This week was really tough. It's okay to give in to the urges. It will make you feel better.* I was nowhere close to being cured.

In medical school, you spend the first two years in the classroom, trying to stay awake while listening to endless lectures. You spend the second two years rotating through medical and surgical specialties, trying to stay awake despite sleep deprivation and standing as still as a statue during eight-hour surgeries, all while figuring out what you want to do for the rest of your life. No pressure. Sitting in a classroom with my nose buried in a textbook turned out to be the easy part.

In the hospital, we were expected to do the grunt work of everyone above us in the hierarchy, including nurses, residents, fellows, and attending physicians. Sometimes we were their scribes; sometimes we fetched coffee; other times, we held surgical tools for hours until our fingers fell asleep. We followed so closely on our superiors' heels that on occasion we came embarrassingly close to following them into the bathroom stall. We ran around the hospital at all hours of the day and night; we were expected to be on overnight call and get in at 4 a.m. like surgery residents but without the authority to actually treat patients. It was all part of the learning experience, but it seemed more like fraternity hazing—instead of getting drunk, we disimpacted the rectums of constipated patients.

I was scared away from some specialties—even an entire semester of anatomy lab couldn't steel me for the savagery of an operating room—and gravitated toward others, like neurology and psychiatry. In class, we learned about neurotransmitters and how they could affect mood and behavior; too many or too few could tip the mental health seesaw into full-blown mental illness. Then I saw the science play out in real time as I spent four weeks on the inpatient adult psychiatric unit. Every time I entered the unit, the loud click of the automatic locks on the doors reminded me that I was easily entering a place that was much harder to leave—a place where people were kept involuntarily because they needed saving and they could no longer save themselves.

Some of the severely depressed patients were immobilized by catatonia and stripped of their short-term memory by electroconvulsive therapy (ECT), a treatment that was supposed to make them better. The schizophrenic patients hallucinated, reaching for imaginary things on the ceiling and picking at their skin as if it were covered with bugs. And then there was the young woman with bulimia, swallowed up in baggy clothes, her arms wrapped tightly around her body, looking sad and avoidant. I was told to interview her and report back to the attending psychiatrist on rounds.

"Good morning. How are you doing today?" I asked, introducing myself as a third-year medical student, in case she couldn't tell by the short white coat and giant pocket guide to all things medical weighing me down. "I'm okay," she replied, avoiding eye contact. "Did you have any trouble sleeping last night? How is your appetite?" I asked. *I could be you*, I thought. *You can talk to me.* I wished she could receive my telepathic messages. It was my job to sit there with my pencil and notepad like a journalist, to sit through whatever awkward silence, tangential thoughts, or paranoia a patient shared with me. I was no therapist, and yet I had to ask her invasive questions about her illness, about childhood traumas that could have led to her eating disorder.

Was she sexually or physically abused when she was younger? Did her parents shame her into losing weight? *Was it any of my business?* I understood her struggle, constantly torn between wanting to be healthy and relapsing into self-destructive behaviors. But we were on opposite sides of the glass, and I imagine it felt to her more like an interrogation than an interview. That afternoon I ran until I forgot about the interview, forgot that it could just as easily be me in that psych unit, hugging my knees to my chest and waiting to escape.

I wanted so badly to run away from my demons. I could not outrun them metaphorically, but I started to wonder if I could outrun them physically. Running was a powerful mental distraction, more potent than the painting and meditation I had done in group therapy. When I was running, thoughts of bingeing never crossed my mind. Running and bingeing were diametrically opposed, healthy against unhealthy, sane against insane, movement against inertia. If I wanted to be healthy, I had to commit to running. The Rutgers Unite Half Marathon was my opportunity to go from non-runner to runner.

In the middle of half-marathon training, Ken broke up with me, nearly derailing my progress. He blamed the breakup on medical school: I was too busy for him; I would never have time for a family. Drive and ambition, traits he once admired about me, were now my inadequacies. It hurt like hell to have my strengths hurled back at me as weaknesses. Five years after our relationship began, it was over. I was devastated, but I refused to apologize for following my dreams, and decided to use my pain and anger to energize my runs.

    I kept training, slowly increasing my miles on the treadmill, running up to 8 to 10 miles at a time. I wasn't fast, but I was persistent, keeping the pace around ten minutes per mile. I felt ready. On the day of the race, it was amazing to push myself to 13.1 miles, the longest distance I had ever run in a single effort. The Rutgers Unite race weaved around my campus and cut through Johnson Park, making it feel familiar and conquerable. I kept a steady pace through Johnson Park, climbed over the bridge that crossed the Raritan River, and jogged down George Street all the way to downtown New Brunswick.

    I neared the finish line, where crowds of people urged on the runners amidst the smell of the fried food trucks that were a permanent fixture of Easton Avenue. My mom was there to cheer me on, just as she had been at all my soccer games, taking photos from the sidewalk as I jogged past. Afterward, I collapsed in a heap. I couldn't believe my body had carried me that far, and, for a split second, I wondered if it could go even farther. When my friends asked if I would ever consider a marathon, I firmly replied, "No, only crazy people run marathons. Why would anyone torture themselves by running *26 miles??*" I thought I knew it all then; a half-marathon was hard, and I was wise to spare myself from anything worse. Little did I know I was only a few years away from running marathons and more.

Chapter 8

THE INVISIBLE MONSTER

I lived my twenties in four-year epochs, punctuating them with graduations and moves from one school or town to the next. At twenty-six, I made my biggest move yet to the gritty, bustling city of Philadelphia. After graduating from medical school, the initials MD were a nominal achievement stamped on a paper certificate; technically, I was a doctor, but I could not practice medicine until I completed a residency. It felt like being told I could play in the soccer game and then having to watch from the sidelines.

During my clinical rotations, I had fallen in love with neurology. I was fascinated by the way the brain worked; diagnosing neurologic disorders was not unlike piecing together a 1,000-piece jigsaw puzzle, and I happened to be good at puzzles. My choice of specialty bound me to four to six more years of training before I would have a *real* job.

The walk from the hospital to home was only four blocks, but on the toughest days, it felt like four miles. When I wasn't dead tired, I liked strolling along Walnut Street, perusing shop windows and inhaling the aromas coming from its innumerable coffee shops, restaurants, and food trucks. There were so many things to see in such a short distance; every block held something new, and city life felt exciting. But when exhaustion set in, the city's flaws overtook its beauty: Each crack in the sidewalk was magnified. Every garbage can teemed with an overwhelming stench. The bleak, monochromatic buildings, tall and imposing, were indifferent to the struggles of people living on the streets. My Skechers seemed glued to the sticky asphalt as if they were melting with each sluggish step.

I opened the door to my third-floor studio apartment, threw my bag on the floor, and collapsed on the bed. The air conditioner unit on the wall whined with exertion, trying to fight the stifling 100-degree heat of late summer. Another long day in the emergency room, and I was beat. The ER was full of outrageous cases—everything from patients vomiting blood, foreign bodies in surprising places, and hideous abscesses needing to be drained, to intoxicated patients bursting out of four-point restraints and swinging at the staff and security. Before I could get anywhere near the neurology wards and start my specialty training, the first year of residency was spent rotating through internal medicine and all its subspecialties, which included the chaotic ER at Thomas Jefferson University Hospital.

Residency was medical school in overdrive. Residents were paid, but the pay was meager compared to the heaping $300,000 in student debt most of us had accumulated. Residents were doctors and students at the same time, with our ability to write orders, prescribe medication, and treat patients overshadowed by the fear and anxiety of making mistakes when we weren't being supervised. When not taking care of patients, we presented at case conferences, listened to lectures, and studied. It was a blur of lengthy workweeks—sometimes stretches of fourteen or more days in a row—made up of twelve- to fourteen-hour shifts, overnight calls, and too many cups of coffee in a fast-paced hospital environment. Time lost all meaning until that one "golden weekend" of the month when we had two full days off, which usually meant two full days of hibernating in our studio apartments in a daze of post-call fatigue.

We were expected to learn and work efficiently and to stay smart and sharp even when sleep-deprived. We were lucky, the attending physicians said, to have eighty-hour workweeks; it was much harder "back in the day." On rounds, they battered us with any esoteric medical question of their choosing, at any moment. "List all the components of the extrinsic and intrinsic coagulation cascade." "Interpret this EKG." "What are the urea cycle disorders that cause hyperammonemia?" From hematology to cardiology to nephrology, the questions bounced from organ system to organ system. It was embarrassing to not know the answer, and even worse to be one-upped by the next resident who answered correctly.

Needless to say, the stress of residency far surpassed anything I had ever faced before. When the first coffee of the day wore off, I found myself reaching into the pockets of my white coat, hungry after working for four hours straight. It was only 9 a.m. Granola bars, graham crackers, and candy bar wrappers brushed up against my stethoscope, which had touched countless patients' gowns and bare skin. But I didn't care: I needed a snack. I was too busy worrying about my patients' health to worry about my own, too tired from walking the halls of the hospital to walk to the grocery store. Baggy hospital scrubs masked the weight I had gained from stress eating and snacking from the vending machine at odd hours of the day, the doctor's version of the "freshman fifteen."

After work, I was listless, and crashing on the bed in the middle of my 400-square-foot studio became a ritual. I missed running. It was cast aside, deprioritized once I became a doctor, like so many other things I once enjoyed. Every day I was faced with the same choice: lie there in a pile, or get up and go outside for a jog? Or, door number 3: go to the corner market, buy as much food as I could carry, and binge the stress away. Every day was a new roll of the dice.

On the days I laced up my sneakers, my headphones drowned out the chaos of Center City, and I momentarily forgot the stress that came with work and my fucked-up relationship with food. Despite the polluted air, frequent stops at traffic lights, and jostling elbows of pedestrians that came with running on busy city streets, I was free. A two-mile run could take me all the way to the banks of the Schuylkill River or across the Benjamin Franklin Bridge, places that felt far away when I was trapped in a cramped apartment. On the days I chose food or sleep, I felt remorse. I had missed an opportunity to make myself healthier. It was a constant battle to find consistency.

The digital display on the treadmill hit 4.97 miles; then 4.98, 4.99, and finally 5.00. That was my trigger to power down the machine and stretch. How had I ever run 13.1 miles? I blotted my face with a towel; the whir of the fans mitigated some of the stuffy air inside, but I was sweating profusely. A twenty-dollar monthly membership at the gym on Walnut Street was all I could afford with my resident salary. Every bag of groceries, every drink at the bar was calculated into my budget. And I wasn't about to waste twenty hard-earned dollars.

I started building in daily treadmill runs, mechanically checking off three to five miles, stopping as soon as I hit the planned distance for that day. The gym kept me accountable, and the treadmill took away the obstacles of running outside. I was running to burn calories and get fit, but I was also trying to make it a habit. At the time, I realized that I needed to replace bad habits with good ones, but I did not realize how critical that concept would be to my recovery. Exercising was a good habit, but one of the hardest ones to form. It required time and dedication, things that felt scarce outside the hospital.

"I saw you running this morning at 6 a.m. when I was walking to work," my friend Anna texted. "You're crazy!" She didn't know that running was actually making me *less* crazy. Once it became a part of my routine, I was determined to stick with it. It grounded me. When Anna saw me out for a morning jog, I had just come off an overnight shift. I had run around the hospital all night from one emergency to the next, listening to the dyssynchronous beeping of seven pagers bouncing around on the waistband of my scrub pants, answering the calls of nurses and patients. It was the fourth night of a three-week stretch of night float.

Sometimes there was a lull around 2 a.m. and I napped, only to be awoken by shrill beeping minutes later, but for the most part, I was awake all night and had only a handful of hours to sleep during the day before the next onslaught. But running through the city at 6 a.m. was enticing. The city had yet to wake from its overnight slumber, and the streets were peaceful and quiet as the light of dawn started to filter over the roofs of the high-rise buildings. I could run without bumping into anyone; I could hear my own breath and focus my thoughts. I was alone in a city of millions.

Friendships in residency were like friendships in medical school—forged quickly and through mutual suffering. Even if you had nothing else in common, you knew what it was like to be awake for thirty-six hours. I bonded with Anna during my internal medicine year, and she became one of my best friends; she even understood when I missed her wedding, stuck working in the medical ICU as she walked down the aisle. But despite our close friendship, she knew nothing of my eating disorder. I kept it secret, confined to the walls of my shabby apartment. The bulimia was invisible to everyone around me, including the people I spent the most time with over the following three years: my neurology co-residents.

Collectively, we were the biggest nerds in the hospital, with ophthalmoscopes, reflex hammers, and tuning forks banging around in our white coat pockets as we ran to stroke alerts and stat consults. Most of us wore eyeglasses, and some of the guys wore bow ties. But we were respected; there was a healthy fear of neurology among other specialties in the hospital, and they relied on us to give astute recommendations. *The patient won't wake up? Can't move their right arm? Can't speak? Call neurology.* Being a neurologist made it okay to be a nerd for the first time in my life.

With my neurology co-residents

My co-residents were my work family, a tight-knit group of eight men and women who worked feverishly as a team on the wards. As second-year residents, every night we passed the baton of overnight call, which meant covering the neuro ICU, the epilepsy unit, the ER, and the neurology ward for fourteen hours straight. Those patients were *sick*. We looked out for each other. We made each other laugh when we felt like crying. We went out to the bar after work and drowned our sorrows in alcohol. We won as a team, and we lost as a team.

"Starbucks for lunch again?" Sana teased as we sat down for noon lecture on Monday. "How many lattes can you drink in one day?" I laughed and brushed off her comment, joking about my love of coffee as a justification for drinking it all day. She loved coffee too. It was hard not to be a Starbucks addict with a store on every city block. Her comment was harmless, and she had no idea that my choice of coffee was deeply pathologic. My eating disorder—the invisible monster—was telling me to fast that day. I needed to detox from another weekend of indulgence, and I felt completely incapable of making healthy food choices. I could not trust myself around food.

I wasn't the only one who wanted to let loose after a long week of work, and Saturday night had been spent in a comfy booth at El Vez, one of our favorite Mexican restaurants. Aside from good food, they were famous for their Pink Cadillac margaritas, and we wasted half our paychecks refilling the pitcher. We rolled around in laughter, talking over the volume of the busy bar, piling into the photo booth to take group pictures. The table was littered with leftover chips, quesadillas, and shot glasses. We had so much fun that the night spilled over into a bar on Fifteenth Street and didn't end until 3 a.m. I had to be back to work again at five, ready to see all the ICU patients before rounds began at eight. "Work hard, play hard" was the mantra of the resident doctor.

I sipped my skinny vanilla latte and glanced up at the screen at the head of the conference room. It was a drawing of the brain, divided neatly into brightly colored amorphous segments known as Brodmann areas—all fifty-two of which I had committed to memory like a poker player counting cards. There was Broca's area, involved in expressive language; the primary visual cortex, essential to the processing of visual stimuli; the primary motor cortex, integral to the execution of voluntary movements. Part of the puzzle of neurologic diagnosis was correlating physical and mental symptoms with dysfunction in discrete areas of the brain. When a stroke or brain tumor obliterated one region, the patient's symptoms could tell you where the problem was located before an MRI could.

There was no area of the brain labeled "eating disorder." I wished there were, so I could blame my problems on the dysfunction of one self-contained part of my brain rather than a mess of disordered circuitry. I would scour it with a stainless-steel sponge or burn it to ashes with a match. There were neurosurgeries that aimed to do just that, to burn out the circuits involved in eating disorders, but I was not willing to be an experimental lab rat. There was no simple answer to my problem.

While the wild nights and weekends with my work family were fun and exciting, my life became a ping-pong game of excessive partying at night and long shifts in the hospital during the day. The loss of control sent me into a spiral of negative thoughts and emotions, and the bulimia followed suit; I was hydroplaning, with no choice but to steer into the crash. My attitude toward food shifted from week to week, day to day, even hour to hour. I couldn't seem to get it right.

Somewhere within me, I knew I was letting the eating disorder win. Running was a temporary reprieve, but all too often I skipped the run and chose to follow my bad habits. I gave in to bingeing and purging behaviors more than I ever had before, sometimes two or three times a day. The urges felt more powerful than gravity, pulling me down deeper.

I showed up for work every day looking professional and well put together, engaged in my job. On morning rounds, I buried any thoughts of my inner demons. Somehow, despite my mental illness, I was thriving as a resident. I was given an award for clinical excellence on the neurology wards, a plaque mounted on my wall to remind me I was a good doctor. Then the residency program director approached me after morning conference. "We'd like to make you a chief resident for your senior year," he said, extending a congratulatory handshake before I had even accepted. He knew it was an honor I couldn't refuse. I was still Little Miss Perfect in the eyes of my peers and my mentors. They put me up on a pedestal, while I felt as low as a barnacle clinging to a sunken ship. *How am I continuing to achieve these things?* I thought. I didn't know how my brain had the capacity to juggle so much. *Can't these people see how flawed I am?*

I stood at my patients' bedsides with their families and wondered if they could see a scarlet letter instead of a hospital logo stitched onto the lapel of my white coat. Did they know I was a fraud? Doctors were supposed to lead by example, to be a symbol of health and strength for their patients. The patients on the neurology ward were severely disabled by illnesses that took away their ability to walk, make decisions, or speak for themselves. And there I was, standing tall, flashing a smile that exuded confidence, and I felt like a liar. I was a hypocrite—no better than an obese bariatric surgeon or a chain-smoking pulmonologist; I was the neurologist who had lost her mind. In front of patients who had lost their youth, their health, and their dignity, I was squandering mine on a path of self-destruction.

I was stuck in a cycle of fasting then bingeing, running then stagnating, achieving then failing. It was a twisted merry-go-round, spinning faster and faster, and I struggled to hold on to the safety bars. It was only a matter of time before I was thrown off and pulled beneath the platform. I needed to scrub speed, and the brake came at the end of the most shameful night of my life.

I was too excited about going out, unsure if my fingertips were trembling from anticipation or low blood sugar as I applied eyeliner and blush. My mind, like my right hand holding the mascara brush, felt wobbly and unsteady. My thoughts raced, and every emotion seemed heightened. Was I bulimic, or bipolar? My wild behaviors and impulses were taking on a life of their own.

The night started out with not one but two dates, both ending in sex. Was that too wild? For a single person living in a city, maybe not. By 10 p.m., I had come home and changed into a black dress, touched up my makeup, and headed out to the bar with my co-residents as if nothing had happened. I threw back shot after shot of vodka until my vision blurred, and I staggered as I hit the dance floor. That didn't stop me from recklessly dancing and entertaining my friends with my drunken sloppiness. I was the life of the party, ready to do anything and everything that night. If they had told me to steal a car or start a bar fight, I would have. When I became too drunk to walk home, my friends helped me back to my apartment door. But my night didn't end there. Disinhibited from the alcohol, I gave in to a relentless bingeing and purging episode.

The next morning, I woke up in a slumped pile on the bathroom floor, a toothbrush dangling from my hand and the smell of the bar emanating from my crumpled dress. My breath reeked of alcohol and sugar, the dusty remnants of a powdered donut at the corner of my lips. I had never even made it to my bed, and it was time to go back to work. I looked in the mirror, expecting to see the demon with the bloodshot eyes glaring at me, the one that came over me in the throes of a binge. But instead, I just saw myself, with smudges of mascara and dried tears on my cheeks. I was fucking pathetic.

Inertia glued me to the floor as a fresh wave of tears poured out. I felt more than shame or guilt that morning; I felt *hate*. I had never hated anyone—I didn't hate my dad for leaving us, I didn't hate my ex-boyfriend for not knowing how to fix me, I didn't hate the therapists who told me what was wrong with me—but I hated myself in that moment. *Slut. Fat. Worthless. Disgusting.* Brutal words filled my mind and made my chest ache—words so heavy that I could hang them up on the wall next to my awards and diplomas. How could someone who had achieved so much think so little of herself? My hangover was both physical and emotional, but the shame of my actions would take longer to wear off than the alcohol would.

As it turned out, that moment was exactly what I needed to see the truth. Sometimes you need to hit rock bottom to see the blue skies above you. Anorexia was my quest toward perfection, which is why I never wanted to be cured of it. But bulimia had invaded my mind like a toxin, making my skin crawl with shame and self-loathing. It was not welcome. And it was not *me*. Maybe I didn't need to be perfect, but I needed to be okay. Somewhere within me was still a *good* person, with a good heart and good intentions; I just had to find her. I needed to get rid of the poison and reset my mind. Then the universe granted me a gift: the chance to find myself again far, far away in the Rocky Mountains.

Chapter 9

PRACTICE MAKES PERFECT

The first time I binged in college, I was surprised and horrified, but I shouldn't have been. My body *needed* food. And it needed a *lot* of food to rebound to a normal weight. Up to 85 percent of people with anorexia will end up binge eating at some point. This can be an adaptive response to starvation regardless of the cause—poverty, war, neglect, self-induced starvation, or in the case of the Minnesota study, the result of an experiment that toys with levels of serotonin and dopamine in the brain.

Binge eating can also be a response to food insecurity. According to a *Current Psychiatry Reports* review, food insecurity in young adults has been associated with depression, anxiety and eating disorders, especially binge eating.[20] Individuals living with food insecurity go through feast-or-famine cycles in which food intake fluctuates with food availability, decreasing during periods of scarcity and increasing during periods of abundance. This might look like waiting for monthly food stamps or a child support payment, then splurging on a trip to the grocery store. For me, it was relying on my mom's under-the-table cash when she cleaned houses and creating as many unpalatable dinners from canned vegetables as possible, then, when I moved to college, having unlimited access to food—the unhealthy kinds of foods that appeal to binge eaters and college students alike. I packed on pounds faster than you could say Entenmann's.

If it was true that my body simply needed to gain weight, then surely my binge eating should have stopped when I returned to a normal weight, right? Wrong. It was too late to stop the behavior; it had become a habit.

Habits

Let's go back to the limbic system, the primitive part of the brain (the downstairs of our two-story house) that spurs adolescent urges and actions before the prefrontal cortex has fully developed. The limbic system plays a pivotal role in emotion, learning, memory, fight-or-flight responses, and maintaining homeostasis. It is one of the oldest parts of the brain, common to fish, amphibians, reptiles, and the mammals that came before us. It is also incredibly complex, situated deep within the brain and composed of so many discrete structures and interrelated parts that even neurology residents can't memorize it. We dreaded being tested on it.

Two of the most important areas are the hippocampus, involved in learning and memory, and the amygdala, which is involved in emotional regulation and response, especially in regard to fear. When you see a snake on the ground, the amygdala tells you to scream and jump away from it, before the rest of your brain realizes it is just a tree branch. The limbic system also includes the hypothalamus, the control center that regulates the endocrine, or hormonal, system—the same area that stopped me from getting a period when I was too thin. Dysfunction of the limbic system occurs in patients with epilepsy, dementia, autism, bipolar disorder, and schizophrenia, to name a few conditions. For people with binge eating disorder and bulimia, the most important parts of the limbic system are the nucleus accumbens, the reward center of the brain that we discussed earlier, and the basal ganglia, which is a group of gray matter nuclei involved in voluntary motor movements, pattern recognition, learning, and habit formation.

Your brain can take any routine activity and turn it into a habit, good or bad. This includes actions like flossing your teeth every day, drinking coffee first thing in the morning, or biting your nails. It also includes things like snorting cocaine or watching porn. There's a fine line between a bad habit and an addiction; the former can quickly turn into the latter when it is done regardless of the negative consequences.

The limbic system does not discriminate between good and bad; its function is merely to speed up the process of habit formation. Some studies say it takes weeks or months to form a habit, but every person is different, and as with nature versus nurture, there are many factors that play a role. But in the end, it boils down to four essential steps, deeply rooted in the limbic system: cue, craving, response, and reward.

The first time I binged, my brain was triggered by food. Not just any food, but a large amount of food rich in sugar and fat: a freshly baked Funfetti cake with gooey vanilla icing and sprinkles. That was the cue. My brain recognized a potential reward: a stomach full of delicious cake. Smelling the cake and feeling my stomach grumble produced craving. A surge of dopamine was released in anticipation of the reward. My response was both mental and physical: debating if I should eat the cake, then giving in, picking up a fork, and savagely digging into it.

That was the first time I gave in to the craving. The reward was obvious: My nucleus accumbens lit up like a string of holiday lights in response to so much decadent food. That cake was delicious, and I needed more of it.

In the brains of people without eating disorders, this process would not be much different in response to foods like pizza, chocolate, or a cheeseburger; food is a powerful motivator and reward, and we all get cravings. Food also stimulates opioid receptors, the same receptors involved in addiction to substances like fentanyl and oxycontin, as I will discuss later.

In my brain, the process went haywire. The nucleus accumbens told the hippocampus and the amygdala to *remember* how great the food tasted and how happy I felt while I was eating it, and to prompt me to seek it out again. It also communicated with the basal ganglia, telling it to pay attention so it would *learn* the behavior, in case it might be used again in the future. All these areas continued to chatter back and forth excitedly about what I had just done. My brain completed this complex circuit of communication with lightning speed, without my conscious awareness or permission.

The next time I binged, my brain completed the circuit a little bit faster. And then faster. And faster. It became extremely efficient at it, until a "moment of weakness" or a "cheat day" turned into habitual bingeing. My limbic system became adept at sending me signals, which I identified as urges, to repeat the behavior and binge again, seeking the same reward. Every time I gave in to the urges, it strengthened the signaling loop. It turned a rubber band into a steel cable.

The stronger this signaling loop became, the less energy I needed to spend on maintaining my habit. This happened through a process called neuroplasticity, which is the ability of neural networks to change through growth and reorganization. Our thoughts, experiences, and actions can transform the way our brains are wired and impact how much of our brain function is dedicated to specific tasks. Habits put our brain on autopilot, thus requiring less energy and attention to perform the habit. And when it gets easier and easier to perform a habit, it gets harder and harder to change it.

Learning

A key part of learning a habit is memory, and the hippocampus plays an integral role in memory formation. When people think of memory, they usually think of explicit memory, or the conscious recollection of facts or experiences—memorizing the US presidents in chronological order in fifth grade, or recalling the name of the first music album you bought as a teenager. But there is also implicit memory, which involves nonconscious learning of skills, habits, and other behaviors. Classic examples include learning to ride a bike or throw a baseball. We can go years without using those skills, but we still know how to do them when we decide to pedal down the road on a spring day or toss a baseball around in the backyard.

The more often a behavior or routine is practiced, the easier it becomes to perform, because it becomes a part of implicit memory. The brain does not care if we remember how to do things correctly or perfectly; it just remembers that we did them. Instead of "practice makes perfect," it's really "practice makes permanent." It is much harder to get rid of implicit than explicit memory; for instance, when someone has amnesia after a traumatic brain injury, it is often the explicit memories that are affected, not the implicit ones. Old habits die hard.

The best learning, memorizing, and habit formation takes

place when we are young, when the limbic system dictates how we behave. If we learn to set an alarm clock and make the bed every day as a kid, we will likely do those things as an adult. If we never learn the habit of chewing with our mouth closed, chances are we will have bad table manners forever. It might not be impossible, but it is difficult to teach an old dog new tricks.

Because habit formation and addiction are closely linked, adolescence is again a vulnerable period for the brain, just as it is with eating disorders. By twelfth grade, 50 percent of teens have tried illicit drugs at least once, and 62 percent have used alcohol. Early substance use correlates with substance abuse problems later in life, and the chance of developing an addiction is five times greater when substance use begins in the teen years as opposed to the twenties. Addictions, like other habits, stick in young minds.

Conditioning

To add another layer of complexity, our brains make associations that can strengthen habits and memories. This is called classical conditioning, which you might know as Pavlovian conditioning. Ivan Pavlov, a Russian physicist, first discovered this phenomenon when studying the digestive process of dogs. Pavlov noticed that his dogs would salivate any time they were given food, which is a normal innate response—in other words, an unconditioned response—for a hungry animal. Every day he fed his dogs following a routine: first opening the door to the lab, then pushing the food in on a cart, and then presenting the food. Over time, he noticed that the dogs would start salivating any time the cart was brought in, before the food was presented to them; that is, they were responding to an *unrelated* stimulus.

9 | PRACTICE MAKES PERFECT

To test this further, he paired the presentation of food with a bell. The bell in this case was a conditioned stimulus, a cue that was not inherently related to the food at all, but one that signaled a reward was coming. He would ring the bell, then feed the dogs. Over time, the dogs began to salivate when the bell rang—*before* they saw the food—because they associated the bell with being fed. Essentially, Pavlov showed that a behavior could be triggered without the primary stimulus—in this case, food—even being present. However, when he continued to ring the bell *without* feeding them, the behavior extinguished, or resolved. That is, once the reward was taken away, the dogs stopped responding to the cue. Pavlov's work has been used in addressing many mental health disorders in treatments such as aversion therapy and exposure therapy, which help extinguish habits and fears. It also played a huge part in my recovery from bulimia.

Classical conditioning is everywhere. Picture a smoker who lights a cigarette whenever they drink a cup of coffee. Coffee doesn't affect their desire to smoke, but conditioning does. The coffee is an associated trigger, just like a fifteen-minute work break or eating a meal might be. Similarly, for a drug addict, the cues might not be the drug itself, but rather the things that surround the drug use: the same apartment, the same group of people, the music playing at the party. Associations can be positive or negative, depending on how our brains remember them. Think of the last time you were sick with the flu, and the last thing you ate before you got sick—maybe a plate of scrambled eggs. After that experience, you might never eat eggs again—because of that memory, even the smell of them in a diner might make you nauseous. The scrambled eggs did not *cause* the illness, but they are negatively *associated* with it.

For me, there were many cues to binge that had nothing to

do with food, things that set the stage for gluttony. Stress was a big one, as was being alone. My brain was even conditioned to certain smells, like the scented candles on the coffee table in my studio apartment. The limbic system loves to attach memory and emotional resonance to scents. My limbic system, the origin of my urges, used these cues as kindling to light a burning fire within my mind, one that I could not put out until I binged. *You had a long, stressful day at the hospital. Eating will make you feel better,* it prodded me. *No one is here with you. No one will know.* It was telling me lies. While eating large amounts of food was rewarding for a few minutes, it was followed by compensatory purging and feelings of guilt and shame. But my limbic system paid no mind to that. Once the fire was lit, it continued to rage.

The Inner Voice

The average human brain has about six thousand thoughts per day. A fair number of them are intrusive thoughts—thoughts that are irrelevant, nonproductive, and sometimes alarming or frightening when they cross our minds. Pushing an old person in front of a bus, jumping off a cliff when you're standing at the edge, hurting an animal or baby. For most people, these thoughts are not aligned with our true desires, and we usually brush them away, knowing we are good people and would never do such terrible things.

But in the mind of someone with an eating disorder, post-traumatic stress disorder (PTSD), obsessive-compulsive disorder (OCD), or body dysmorphic disorder, intrusive thoughts are harder to ignore. They morph into urges and obsessions intricately linked with our habits. In the case of OCD, the response to an intrusive thought can become a ritual, or compulsion, a series of actions done to lessen the anxiety that comes with an obsession. A perceived fear of contamination, from someone else's germs or touching a surface that appears dirty, might lead to excessive handwashing, showering, cleaning, or throwing out anything that might be contaminated. Sometimes complex rituals cannot completely resolve the fear, and that person still might lose sleep over it. But attempting to suppress obsessive thoughts and not respond to them only makes those thoughts more intense and persistent.

In the formation of habits or addictions, cues are only as meaningful as we allow them to be. That's why it is so alarming when an inner voice tells you to binge eat or drink a bottle of vodka or check all the light switches in your house ten times. Many people with bulimia identify their urges to binge as an inner voice that is not so different from their own. Some anthropomorphize their urges, giving them proper names, like Sally Sweet Tooth or Becky Binge. Some nicknames are made to sound humorous or harmless, the same way drug users refer to meth as "cotton candy" or heroin as "brown sugar." But there are also less friendly nicknames—the Bitch, the Monster, the Demon—that denote how sinister the urges can sound. For me, the urges were anxiety-producing and unwelcome. The voice was my own, but it did not align with my true sense of self.

I didn't realize until I was a neurologist, and fully recovered from my eating disorder, that the monster telling me to binge was actually my limbic system. It drove the cues and the cravings that I couldn't ignore. Like dopamine, the limbic system plays an important role in survival, but it can also be the villain in the setting of neuropsychiatric illness—the source of psychotic symptoms following an epileptic seizure, the origin of violent flashbacks in PTSD, or the warped clock on the wall that confuses time and disorients the mind of a patient with dementia.

Once I recognized the power my limbic system had over me, I knew how to conquer it. My prefrontal cortex, the voice of reason, restraint, and determination—my *true* inner voice—could become the hero of the story. All it had to do was break the worst habit I had ever formed.

Chapter 10

THE MOUNTAINS ARE CALLING

Morning sunlight streamed over the Rockies, illuminating patches of snow that had yet to melt beneath the powerful sun and rising temperatures in Colorado. It was going to be a hot day, but the morning air felt crisp as I stood on my balcony drinking a cup of coffee. Far in the distance, hot air balloons were taking flight near the Flatirons, decorating the sky with pops of color in checkers and stripes.

I looked down at my ceramic mug with the words "Shoot for the moon; even if you miss, you'll land among the stars" on it. That was exactly what I intended to do as I started fresh in a new place. The smell of coffee and the view of the mountains energized me for another day of unpacking. I had arrived in Denver two days earlier, and I was eager to unpack as fast as I could; all I wanted to do was get in my car and drive straight toward the mountains, where beautiful hiking trails and dense groves of pine trees awaited.

My life as a student was over. After four years of college, four years of medical school, four years of residency, and a fellowship in vascular neurology, I was about to start a real job as a neurologist. I was thirty-one years old. Other people my age had already married, bought houses, and had kids, and some had even divorced; I was lagging behind in adulthood because I had married my career. It was time for a big move; instead of crossing the Delaware River, I wanted to cross time zones. I was ready to travel, to see more than I had seen out the backseat window of my parents' station wagon on road trips. When I flew to other cities for medical conferences and residency interviews, I rarely got to explore beyond the lecture hall or the tiny window seat on the airplane.

My friend Katrina knew where to go: Colorado. She and I had spent plenty of time next to each other at our desks in the cramped resident office, working on the clinic and hospital schedules as chief residents, daydreaming about a future beyond Philly. "If I get a job offer, my husband and I are moving out there to hike, and fish, and photograph the Rockies," she said. "You'd probably love it." She was interviewing for a job that was hiring not one, but several new neurologists, and thought it would be a good fit for me. The rest of our bespectacled work family thought otherwise. "Denver's not that great a city. There's nothing to do there." And "I didn't know you liked hiking. You never talk about it." Of course I never talked about it. Residents were corralled into two shared hobbies: talking about how awful residency was, and getting drunk. But I didn't care if Denver lacked the giant skyscrapers that illuminated the East Coast city skylines; it had the backdrop of the mountains.

I flew to Denver for my job interview in March, four months before fellowship graduation. My first trip to Colorado lasted exactly twenty-four hours. Every minute was accounted for:

two direct flights, one night in a basic hotel, a lukewarm continental breakfast, a prepaid ride to the interview. There would be no glamorous Vail resort skiing or five-star restaurants on the company tab. But it didn't matter. I was immediately awestruck by the beauty of the landscape. "Not a bad view from the office, right?" the recruiter asked as we looked at the snowy mountains from the fourth-floor neurology office at Swedish Medical Center. "And when you're not working," he said, "you can go hiking, skiing, ice climbing, camping—anything you want."

Anything I want, I thought as I tried to peel my eyes away from the view. The only mountains I knew were the Appalachians, and they looked like grassy knolls compared to the prominence of the Rockies. The Rocky Mountains were statuesque, solid peaks of granite and dirt, buried beneath feet of snow. I couldn't remember the last time I had seen so much snow. The sun reflected off the pure whiteness that blanketed the mountains so many miles away, and the intensity made my eyes water. Everything in Colorado seemed bolder, brighter, and cleaner than what I was used to on the East Coast. I desperately wanted to go out and explore. If only I had an extra day, or a lifetime. Whatever salary they offered me, the answer was yes.

A few months later, I was planning my cross-country move to Denver. Every signed contract, from relocation to employment, solidified the future and made me impatient. Katrina signed with the same group, and together we counted down the days until the big move. I couldn't wait to get away from Philadelphia. It had started out fun and exciting, but five years later, it was a toxic place for my mental health. It made my eating disorder exponentially worse.

At the fellowship graduation dinner, the attending physicians roasted the fellows. They gave short speeches and handed us gift bags. Some of the gifts were thoughtful, like personalized business card holders, while others were gag gifts. I pulled out a bag of SkinnyPop popcorn, the same snack I brought to noon conference almost every day. It was the way I avoided binge eating while others dug into their cafeteria sandwiches and pizza, and they must have thought it was funny. My cheeks flushed with humiliation. They were poking fun at my pain, expecting me to laugh along with them. I could have told them I was bulimic, demanded an apology, and made them feel like shit for mocking a girl with an eating disorder, but instead I shut my mouth and accepted the gifts, smiling through gritted teeth. I was angry. *Fuck this*, I thought. *I can't wait to get out of here.* If I could have run the mile from the restaurant back to my apartment at that moment, I would have set a personal record.

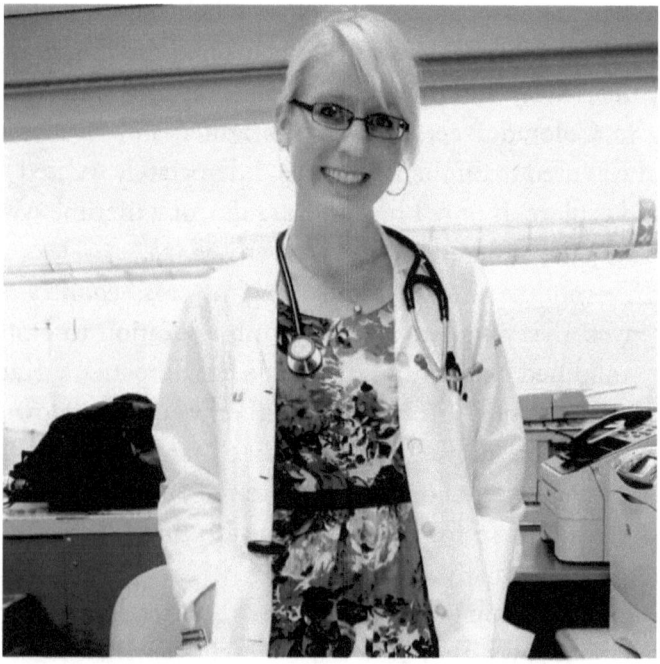

Fellowship in Philadelphia, circa 2016

The growing stack of U-Haul boxes in the corner of my apartment, the farewell dinners with friends and colleagues, the graduation roast. One by one, I untied the knots that tethered me to Philadelphia, so that I could move on to Denver feeling free and unencumbered, ready to start over. I was so close—only six weeks away from moving. And then I met Rich.

He darted from room to room, stretcher to stretcher, intubating, resuscitating, medicating, and calling out orders with a calm confidence. When patients, family members, and nurses panicked, when shit hit the fan, he stayed cool. Nothing seemed to unnerve him, and that was intimidating. But that was what it took to be an ER doctor. He could look relaxed and unflappable while eating a sandwich and charting about bringing the dead back to life, his sneakers and scrubs spattered with bodily fluids. I wasn't sure if that was his personality, or if years of working in the emergency room had hardened him. As he hunched at the computer, the bulging muscles of his back and deltoids strained the seams of his light blue scrub top. He was aloof and almost unapproachable at work, but I quickly found out that beneath that brawny exterior, he was kindhearted and gentle.

I was physically drawn to his bronze skin, dark hair, and umber eyes, the markings of his heritage. He was adopted and brought to the United States just one month after being born in Colombia, a fact that was masked by his adoptive parents' Italian last name and the hint of a New York accent that came out whenever he spoke quickly or excitedly. But I was also drawn to his calm demeanor. I was turbulence, and he was smooth air. Somehow, in five years of working in the same hospital system, we had never meaningfully crossed paths. But once we did, it seemed like there was a magnetic field that kept us drawn to one another. We didn't just connect; we collided, and the impact left us breathless. Two weeks after we met, I told Rich I loved him, and I meant it.

If you believe in destiny, you might know that there are three types of soulmates: a karmic soulmate, a person who enters your life to teach you an important lesson; a companion soulmate, or best friend; and a twin flame, an intense, passionate bond that can only be found with one person in the whole universe. Every day of our relationship was one day closer to moving day, one more grain of sand slipping through the hourglass, and when we weren't together, we sent constant messages and emails. I sent Rich an article about soulmates. "I think you're supposed to be my karmic soulmate," I wrote. "Why else would I meet you right before I move halfway across the country?" His email response was quick and irrefutable. "No. I'm your twin flame." If that was true, then he needed to know the truth about who I was.

We sat at a riverfront table in South Philadelphia, watching the reflection of the clouds in the Delaware River. The waiter placed two glasses of cabernet on the linen tablecloth. It was a romantic spot for lunch, and when he invited me to go, I hadn't hesitated to leave work in the middle of the day. I had one foot out the door already, so close to Colorado, and we were lawless and impulsive. We held hands across the table. No one had ever gazed at me with such intensity. This love was real, more mature than the puppy love I had felt in college. Even though we were still strangers in many ways, I trusted Rich as if I had known him my entire life.

This was my chance, a safe space to share my dark secret. The words started to bubble up, and I couldn't hold them back. "I have to tell you something," I said. My stomach flip-flopped with nerves. Would he let me down like my college boyfriend? Would he ignore my bulimia, or worse, find me ugly because of it? I had a one-way ticket across the country and nothing to lose. Tears pricked my eyes, blurring my vision. "I used to have an eating disorder . . . I mean, I'm still recovering from it. I can't believe I'm telling you this." It was a stretch of the truth. I was still bulimic—I had binged only the day before—but I wanted to believe that I could get better, and saying the words out loud was empowering. I exhaled, feeling lighter. Before he responded, I could see the future with him in it, a life without the shackles that were keeping my mind imprisoned by my eating disorder. He squeezed my hand a little tighter. "Okay. Tell me everything."

I admitted that I was stumbling along a path of attempted recovery and relapses. Some days and weeks were good; some were bad, especially the night I ended up plastered to the tile of my bathroom floor. The fluctuations were as unpredictable as the weather. My attempts at therapy were half-assed at best. I was quick to run away from the feng shui of the therapist's office. I was quick to throw my paintbrush back in the bin, knowing that art would never fully distract me from bingeing; I was left-brained and analytical, not creative enough to be an artist. There was always an excuse, a reason why those therapies wouldn't work for me. In residency, I had tried working to the point of exhaustion, thinking there would be no room left in my tired brain for my eating disorder, and still it managed to consume my every waking thought.

I had even tried to resolve the underlying issue, the root cause that any psychotherapist would point to—my relationship with my dad. Over the years, I had slowly rebuilt a connection with him, first through written letters when he lived across the country in California, then through sporadic visits and phone calls. The relationship would never be perfect, but it was enough to satisfy the need to have both of my parents in my life, a need that never went away as I grew into an adult. I was still angry at him for abandoning us, but the anger waned as the years passed. If a relationship with my dad was what I needed to recover, then everything should have clicked into place and the eating disorder should have vanished. But it never did. The only thing that had ever tempered it was running.

Rich listened to me without judgment. Despite my flaws, he still thought I was beautiful. He looked at me as if I were the North Star, shining bright in an inky black sky. He saw the best version of me, the woman who spoke animatedly about moving to Colorado and exploring the outdoors, as we talked over dinners and glasses of wine and during walks through Washington Square. "You're impossibly attractive," he told me. "The most beautiful woman I've ever met." He said that at the darkest time in my life, when I felt the ugliest. If he could see the lightness and beauty within me, why couldn't I? I wanted to feel as beautiful as he thought I was. I wanted his love, but I also wanted to be able to love myself.

Somewhere along the way, I had lost sight of who I was at the core. When I took the job offer in Colorado, my mom reminded me of my strengths: ambition and perseverance. "You decided you wanted to go to Lehigh, and you made it happen. You decided you wanted to go to medical school, and you made that happen too. Now you want to move across the country to pursue your dreams, and you're doing it. Once you set your mind on something, there is no stopping you," she said. It had been over a decade since my dad left, and thanks to years of therapy and time to heal her heart, she was no longer addicted to alcohol. Her motivational words were back in full force, and I was once again encouraged by them.

She was right. I could do anything I put my mind to. The day before I moved to Denver, I sat in my empty apartment and stared at the flight confirmation on my laptop. Every click of the mouse echoed off the high ceilings, and I was acutely aware of how my life was about to change. The movers had taken all my belongings that morning, except for my scale, which I had thrown in the dumpster.

I was moving across the country by myself to start a new chapter of my life. Colorado was my chance for redemption, my New Year's Day, the Monday of the first week of the rest of my new life. I was ready to use the most powerful tools I had: my drive, my determination, and the ability to grit my teeth and move forward despite any obstacles in my way. I muted everything else and listened to my true inner voice, the one that wanted me to be healthy again. I put faith in the part of my brain that would free me from my eating disorder: the prefrontal cortex. I chose me.

And so I boarded my one-way flight toward the sunny blue skies and mountains of Colorado with a quote fixed in my mind: "Keep your face always toward the sunshine—and shadows will fall behind you." I left the shadows behind. And I quit bulimia.

Chapter 11

RECOVERY IS A MARATHON, NOT A SPRINT

It was the Fourth of July, and the sun scorched the foothills, the gatekeepers to the Rocky Mountains. The heat was abated by the wind, which slammed the car door shut and whipped my hair across my face as I stepped out onto the driveway of a recently built house in Golden. I hated being the new girl, the unfamiliar face at the party, shaking hands and introducing myself over and over. It was exhausting. But these people were approachable and laid-back—a group of doctors, nurses, and their spouses enjoying tacos and cold beers on the wraparound porch—and I would see their faces again in the halls of the hospital.

They didn't care about my resume; there were more interesting things to talk about. How would I spend my first three weeks in Colorado before starting my new job? they asked. Where would I go hiking? The answer was Longs Peak. I was excited to hike in Rocky Mountain National Park, ready to take on my first Colorado "fourteener," a mountain whose summit tops

14,000 feet. The host of the party looked skeptical. "Longs Peak is pretty technical," she said. "How about you try Chasm Lake, halfway to the summit? Let's take a look at a map and I'll show you the route."

I didn't know that Longs Peak was a tough, technical, fifteen-mile hike with significant elevation gain, rock scrambling, and climbing, and only a 50 percent success rate of reaching the summit. I didn't know that when I attempted the climb a few days later in July, in shorts and a T-shirt, a snow squall and freezing temperatures would turn me around before I reached Chasm Lake. I was an amateur—unacclimatized and unprepared. And I was still wearing Asics sneakers; I didn't even own hiking boots yet.

That night I met Danielle, a native Coloradan and ER nurse in one of the hospitals I would be working in. Danielle was tall and lanky with an athletic build, and her outdoor resume was even more impressive than her professional one. Rock climbing, ice climbing, mountaineering, trail running. Like the others at the party, she was interesting and had more to talk about than the daily grind in the hospital. Her life was filled with travel and adventure. She was quietly confident and, like most Coloradans I would meet, friendly and likeable—adjectives rarely used to describe East Coasters. "We should hang out sometime," she said. "Do you want to go for a trail run around Red Rocks?" In Philadelphia, you got to know people over drinks in a crowded bar. In Denver, you had to *move* if you wanted to make friends. Trail running sounded much more challenging than running on flat pavement or the smooth conveyor belt of a treadmill, but I was willing to try. "Sure!" I replied enthusiastically.

I was only four days sober, four days free of bulimia, four days into my new life. No one here knew about my past. Every time I met someone in Colorado, I had the opportunity to show them the person I aspired to be, rather than the ghost I had left behind in Philadelphia. That ghost was now 1,700 miles away. I was determined to become the best version of myself.

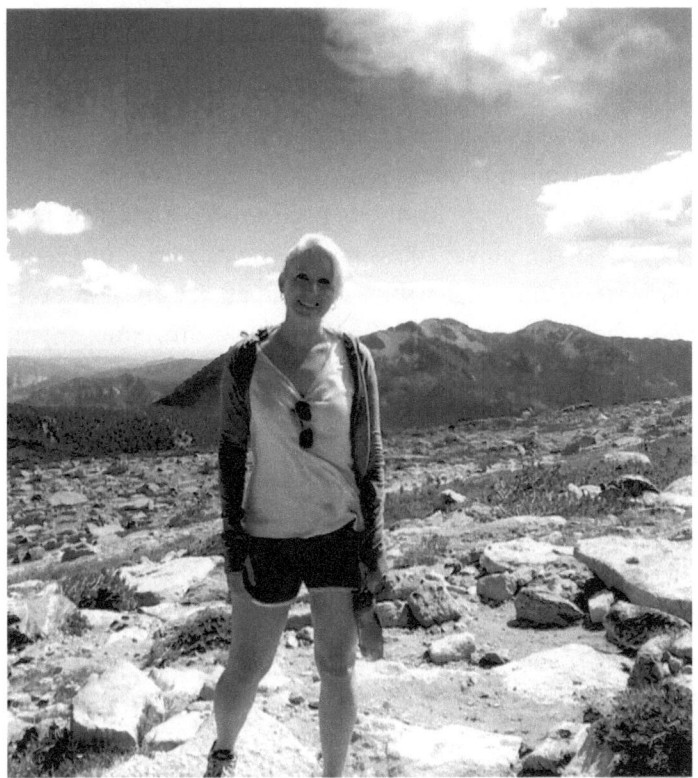

First hike to Chasm Lake

The moment my feet touched the ground at Denver International Airport, I had quit bulimia. I gave it up cold turkey, like an opioid addict throwing away Oxycontin or an alcoholic pouring a full bottle of bourbon down the sink. "Cold turkey," a phrase used today to describe quitting a drug or going through uncomfortable withdrawal symptoms, has an unclear etymology but appears to have been used in the early 1900s as a way to convey the idea of "straightforward," "matter of fact," or "a plain and simple truth." I had finally seen the plain and simple truth as clearly as the blue sky above me: I was addicted to food, but I could choose to stop bingeing and be healthy, just like I had chosen to move across the country.

Buried within any addiction is the ability to make a choice, and that choice comes from our prefrontal cortex. This part of the brain has the power to overcome the primitive urges of the limbic system, to change habits and beat addictions. I didn't have to be a victim, to let the eating disorder destroy me, anymore. The straightforward way to beat my addiction was abstinence—staying as far away from temptation and harmful behaviors as possible. And I would have to make the choice to stay away every day, for as long as it took.

For the first few weeks in Colorado, my addiction followed me like a shadow. The urges came out of nowhere while unpacking boxes, browsing furniture stores, or driving to hospital orientation. They prodded me while I ate dinner on my IKEA sofa; I was at my most vulnerable when I was eating alone. But instead of giving in to the urges, I listened to them and let them pass through my mind. I ignored them. When they got louder and more persistent, I fought back against them in my mind, letting the voice of my prefrontal cortex be my defender. *You're not welcome here. Leave me the fuck alone. I won't give in again.* My prefrontal cortex was the noble, heroic kid fighting back against the bully on the playground. And it was triumphant; one day, months later, the bullying simply stopped.

Withdrawal from addictive substances, both illicit and prescribed, can be uncomfortable, dangerous, and even deadly. But

11 | RECOVERY IS A MARATHON, NOT A SPRINT

when I abruptly stopped binge eating, there was no withdrawal; I felt better *without* it. The effects were both physical and mental. I felt invigorated and alive, like I was waking up for the first time—a bear shaking off the fogginess of hibernation to venture out in the wilderness and morph into a ferocious predator once again. The farther I moved away from the snowy den of mental illness, the clearer my thoughts grew and the more my awareness heightened. I could navigate the world around me with sharper vision and clarity. The pine trees glimmered in vibrant hues of green, shades that had seemed muted before. I was free.

Colorado teemed with things that made me feel alive: sunshine, bright blue skies, breathtaking views of mountains and rivers across a verdant expanse of nature and beauty. It offered plenty of ways to keep my mind distracted from food, to keep my body moving outdoors instead of idling in front of the fridge. Colorado was uplifting, and I could feel it pulling me out of the dysthymia I had settled into for so long.

I spent every weekend visiting a new place with a labyrinth of trails to hike. A solo drive into the mountains was the cure for a long workweek and a way to explore my new surroundings. Even the names of the state and county parks were inviting: Lair o' the Bear, Alderfer/Three Sisters, Golden Gate Canyon, Red Rock Canyon Open Space. After every hike, I came back to my apartment happily spent, with dirty Merrell hiking boots, sun-kissed skin, and stories to share with Rich over lengthy evening phone calls. I missed him terribly, but I loved life in this new place.

Every time I hiked, I immersed myself in the densely forested landscape, and with each breath, I marveled at how clean the air felt. It was thin, dry air, but it no longer made me feel breathless. I didn't realize it at the time, but I had inadvertently started my own biofeedback therapy on those hiking trails; my breathing and heart rate slowed, my muscles relaxed, and my mind was singularly focused on the sounds of nature around me. Instead of music, I listened to the rush of the wind through the subalpine tree line. With nature communicating all around me, talk became superfluous.

The best trails led to mountain lakes, where I kicked off my shoes to stretch my tired legs and sat fixated by the reflection of the mountains in the glassy water. Peanut butter and jelly, the same food that had haunted my dreams when I was anorexic, was now my favorite food on hiking trips. When I was out in nature, nowhere near a fridge, the fear of bingeing did not exist. I could eat one sandwich and feel satisfied after hours of hard hiking. Echo Lake, Odessa Lake, Sky Pond, Emerald Lake—the list grew longer every time I laced up my hiking boots, and my mind started to settle and calm like the lakes' deep blue waters. Colorado was a place for healing.

I was getting a refresher course on the benefits of being outdoors, but a love of nature had always been within me. It started in Blairstown, before my family fell apart, when life was spent playing soccer on freshly cut grass, running around the backyard with my brother and sister, and hiking on the Appalachian Trail. The AT's 2,197-mile course passed almost directly behind my childhood home. During the warm spring and summer months, we walked, ran, or rode our bikes up the gravel road to the Mohican Outdoor Center, a campsite for AT through-hikers. We then hopped onto the trail and traversed the mountain ridge all the way to the Catfish Fire Tower before descending the Rattlesnake Swamp Trail to my mom's parked station wagon, hours away at the next trail junction. As a teenager, the hikes were daylong adventures with my sister or best friend; we would stop to picnic, climb trees, and take pictures of the view with Kodak cameras. Before that, the hikes were with my dad, the expert on all things outdoors. He made nature exciting, showing us how to recognize poisonous plants and use a snakebite kit. Together, we would walk the trail, picking blackberries off their fragrant bushes and dodging the honeybees, the berries ending up in a pie with Mom's buttery homemade crust. Happy memories of the AT filled my mind every time I set foot on a trail in Colorado.

Most of the Coloradans I met loved to hike, but they also liked trail running, rock climbing, backcountry camping, and other activities that were new to me. In Denver, going to an indoor gym was boring; the outdoors was a gigantic natural playground. I listened to stories about ice climbing in Ouray and "peak bagging" all of the fourteeners. Some hikers would "bivvy" overnight with minimal supplies on one summit before moving on to the next, and some even did it during winter for an added challenge. They wore crampons instead of hiking boots. They spoke the language of the mountains, and I once again felt like an eager student. I wanted to be one of them, to learn their dialect. Instead of reading about it in a book, I rented snowshoes, reacquainted myself with skis, and converted my boring treadmill runs into outdoor jogs through city parks and eventually on trails.

If I really wanted to live the healthy lifestyle of a Coloradan, I also had to reacquaint myself with a healthy diet. While not everyone who lived there was a granola-eating hippie, many were. Denver had plenty of vegan and vegetarian restaurants and health food stores. But before I could shop there, I had to unlearn all the useless facts and unfounded ideas about food I had stored in my brain for so many years. "Low-fat" and "diet" labels did not equal "healthy." Coffee was not a meal. Frozen Lean Cuisine meals, although low in calories, were full of salt and unhealthy preservatives. Was it possible to erase the encyclopedia of calorie counts and nutritional information stored in my brain? How could I forget that an egg was 70 calories, or that a two-tablespoon serving of peanut butter was 190 calories? Even if I could not erase those facts, I could choose to ignore them the same way I was ignoring the urges to binge.

It wasn't easy. I was still tempted to eat packaged junk food and frozen dinners after a long day at work. But I started buying foods that I knew were healthy—fish, whole grain bread, fresh vegetables—and cooking in heart-healthy olive oil. At work, I loaded my plate at the salad bar and snacked on fruit and yogurt. The healthier the food, the better I felt after eating it. And feeling good made my new eating habits stick.

Then I returned to something I had abandoned: baking. I missed the joy of licking raw batter off the spoon and tasting banana bread when it was still warm from the oven. This time I baked with real butter—no chalky low-calorie substitutes—and ate what I baked. I taught myself to eat dessert like a normal person again, one piece of cake at a time, and vowed that I would never again deprive myself of the simple pleasures that come with food.

Months later, I found myself near the summit of Pikes Peak. The Pikes Peak Challenge, a fundraising event for the Brain Injury Alliance of Colorado, drew hundreds of hikers to the base of the mountain each year. Standing at 14,115 feet, Pikes Peak is a classic Colorado fourteener, a non-technical hiker's mountain that hovers above the town of Colorado Springs like a rugged, stony deity. I had enjoyed the mountain as a tourist, riding the Pikes Peak Cog Railway on a four-hour journey through bristlecone pine groves and precipitous snowy inclines all the way to the top. I had also driven past it many times on my way to the hospital or to visit the Garden of the Gods. But I had never put my feet on the trail before that day. After acclimatizing to hikes at elevation, I felt up to the challenge.

The hike started at 5 a.m. with headlamps to guide the way.

11 | RECOVERY IS A MARATHON, NOT A SPRINT

We slowly made our way up toward Barr Camp as the luminescent city lights of Colorado Springs faded away with the dawn. With each passing mile, the views became more magnificent, and the smaller, distant peaks below took the shape of rippling waves. Six hours of steady hiking took me from the trailhead to the summit over the course of the thirteen-mile trail.

Near the top, the frigid wind lashed my face and exposed hands, and the temperature plummeted to 39°F. I was not prepared for the cold—it was only September—but there was nowhere to hide. The summit was rocky and steep, without a single tree in sight. Purple flags and mugs of hot chocolate awaited us at the finish line. I felt lightheaded and giddy, a combination of altitude, exhaustion, and the thrill of climbing my first real summit. I was so elated with my accomplishment that I barely noticed the hairy exposed turns of the mountain road as we took yellow school buses back to the base of the mountain. I realized that this endurance event had exceeded the amount of time I had spent running a half-marathon. I started to wonder how much my body was capable of . . .

Back in my apartment, I stood in front of the full-length mirror in my bedroom and studied my reflection—something I hated to do when I was anorexic, when a mirror was a visual reminder that I would never be thin "enough." I was beat. My muscles were sore—the kind of sore that felt oddly good. Dust and dirt coated my calves and Smartwool socks. My skin had a healthy glow from the brilliant rays of Colorado sunshine. I could see the outline of quads beneath the hem of my Adidas shorts, and it reminded me of how strong I felt as a soccer player. For the first time in years, I liked the way I looked. I was fit, not skinny.

I felt beautiful and capable, a size 8, more confident in hiking gear than I had ever been in a dress or white coat. Ironically, I was the same size I had been as a freshman in high school. I had come full circle, after wasting years of my life dieting and obsessing about being thin. My body was an incredible machine, and I had discredited it for so many years. If I could get myself healthy again, if I could summit a fourteener, maybe I could achieve even greater athletic accomplishments. The word "marathon" popped into my head—a word I had previously associated with pain, torture, and misery—but this time it seemed enticing. *Challenge yourself. Maybe it will be the best thing you've ever done.*

I had no idea how to train for a marathon, but I knew it would take discipline, just as medical school and residency had. The official Colorado Marathon in Fort Collins was a few months away, so I printed a sixteen-week marathon training plan and, like a student with a list of homework assignments, started ticking off each workout. Four miles, then six, then ten, with progressively longer weekend runs. The more I ran, the more my muscles got used to long distances. They came to expect constant motion for hours at a time. They pushed a bit farther each time, until I surpassed the half-marathon distance. I was building physical stamina, unaware that I was also building mental stamina.

There were myriad running and biking trails for people who could not escape the city. The High Line Canal Trail, a mostly paved path that wound northeast through the city of Denver and across the Front Range, spanned a total of 71 miles from start to finish. It was the perfect place to train, and I could access it a few miles down the road from my apartment. After a granola bar and a steaming latte with four shots of espresso from my favorite drive-through coffee kiosk, a breakfast essential to my training runs, I set off in my Asics. Even when morning frost clung to the grass, I ran in shorts and let the cold, crisp air prick my thighs until my body warmed up.

Training runs along that path ended up being some of my favorites. The longest runs came with the best sights—ducks swimming across the surface of a nearly frozen lake, an eclipsed view of the Rockies between the trees, prairie dogs popping their heads up from dry dirt fields as I ran by them. The tranquility of the trail outweighed the pain that accumulated in my muscles. As the months progressed, I built my way up to 20 miles, the apex of any marathon training plan.

Sleep was elusive the night before the Colorado Marathon. I lay awake in the hotel room, full of nervous energy. Rich slept soundly next to me, exhausted from his long flight and jet lag. The day started at 4:30 a.m., at which time eight hundred runners were bused up the winding road to the start of the race, 6,000 feet above sea level, deep within the Poudre Canyon. I nodded off as the bus grumbled up the incline for nearly an hour. When we arrived, sunlight was filtering into the canyon, illuminating the uppermost parts of the rock walls, but it had yet to hit the pavement at the starting line. It was a chilly spring morning. I took turns sitting, standing, and stretching, my legs frozen into marble pillars, as I listened to the gentle rush of the river below.

At the starting line, I felt as brave as I did on the first day of medical school when I gripped the scalpel with white knuckles and made the initial cut through preserved skin and fascia. Running a marathon felt monumental. The gun fired, and I took off. The first half of the course was downhill, which seemed like a gift, but eventually every runner's quads would tire from the constant beating. The road hugged the curve of the river through the canyon, and it was blissfully quiet, miles away from the nearest spectator. I felt like I was running as fast as the current, listening to the steady in and out of my breathing and the drumbeat of my sneakers hitting the pavement. There was nothing else to listen to, not even my music playlist, as we were too remote to get a cell signal.

At mile 15, the mouth of the canyon widened and spit out the marathoners. We were back on main roads with cars and spectators. Two miles later, Rich stood on the side of the road, beaming at me. I knew it would hurt to stop and start again, but I braked mid-stride to kiss him and wrap my arms around him. He didn't seem to mind the salty, sweaty embrace. "Why did you stop?!" he asked, surprised. "I didn't think you'd want to lose a second off your race time." But I didn't care about that; I wasn't fast, and I wasn't there to break any records. I was just grateful to see his face. No man before him had ever cheered for me. "I love you," I said, catching my breath. "See you at the finish line!"

Pride and determination coursed through my veins. I had no doubt I would make it to the finish line. I got my legs moving again, first a walk and then a jog, knowing that my strength was waning with the passing of each mile. I passed the 20-mile mark, the formidable "wall" that every marathoner faces, and felt the slow, unrelenting burn of lactic acid building up in my muscles. My legs felt like ship anchors being dragged across the pavement, and my pace slowed despite my brain's telling my legs to keep running; the pain was nothing like I had ever felt before.

But as I kept going, the agony plateaued. *If I can push through this pain*, I thought, *I can do anything*. For all the times I had punished my body with fasting, bingeing, judgment, and self-criticism, it was now proving how strong and tenacious it could be. With only a quarter mile to go, I pushed harder, racing past crowds of people lining the streets of downtown Fort Collins, racing toward the finish line, toward Rich, toward my future as a runner.

11 | RECOVERY IS A MARATHON, NOT A SPRINT

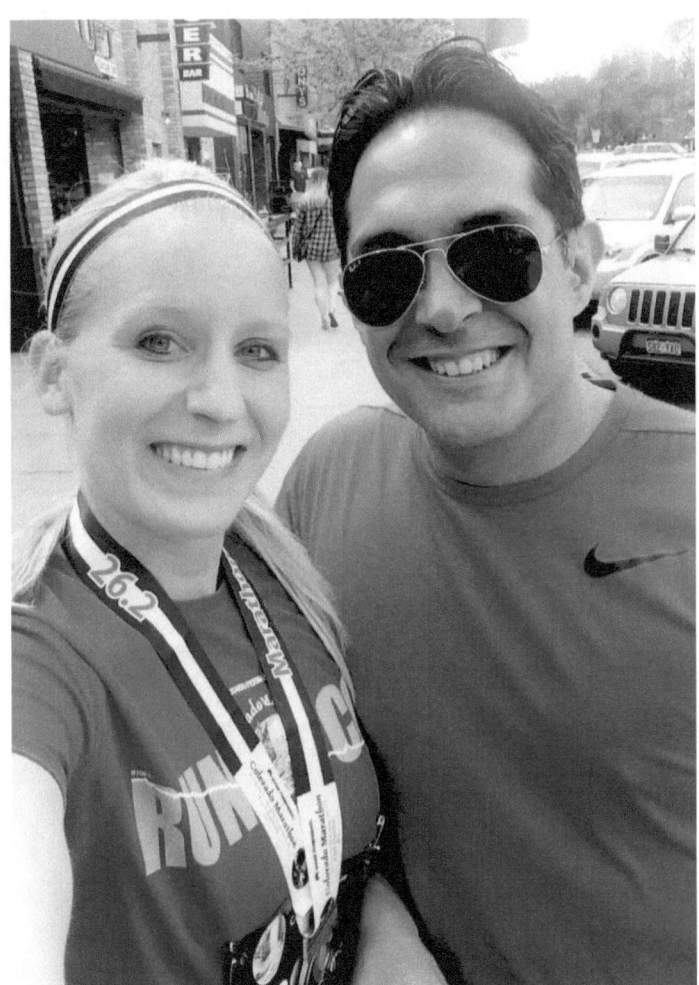

With Rich after the race

Chapter 12

PERFECT MATCH

One year later, I was eager to run the Colorado Marathon again. The weather was just as beautiful, with rays of sunshine beaming down into the canyon. The starting line was exactly where I had left it, the route through the canyon exactly the same. But the race would have a different outcome.

Living in Colorado, I felt healthy again. I was eating right and exercising. Physically, I looked the part of a Coloradan from head to toe—dressed in REI attire and well-worn hiking boots, with blisters on my feet from hiking and running. Mentally, I was free, and my mood was lighter than the hot air balloons that drifted over the Front Range; I did not need a scale to validate that. Best of all, I had not relapsed. Once I saw bulimia as an addiction, the possibility of relapse was always in the back of my mind. Each day of sobriety was a victory. Colorado was my rehab, a safe space, and I never wanted to leave. The only catch was that I loved a man who lived 1,700 miles away, and while he had fallen in love with Colorado too, he was unable to move his entire life there to be with me. I had to choose between the two things I loved most.

I moved back to New Jersey to be with Rich, feeling more anxious than I had felt in a long time. Was it the fear of relapse, or was it being thrown back into suburban hell? Traffic congestion, endless strip malls, cloudy skies, unfriendly faces, and a landscape that looked like it had flatlined. Returning to the East Coast was jarring, all its flaws juxtaposed with the heavenly place I had left behind. The only place I felt relaxed was within the walls of our Cape Cod–style lake house, curled up in the bay window of the kitchen, staring out at the backyard full of rhododendron, oak, and flowering dogwood trees. Rich and I cooked dinners and drank wine in the sunroom of our new house together. It was an oasis amidst the chaos, a place to mourn the loss of the mountains that had restored my health.

I cried over Colorado as if a loved one had passed away. No one understood my grief or the enormity of the loss. "It's just a place," they said. "You can always go back and visit." "Home is where the heart is." But I was not sure where that was anymore. Colorado was not merely a beautiful place to live—it was the place I had found inner peace and healed from my eating disorder. It meant the world to me. I tried to articulate my thoughts, but like a toddler struggling to verbalize the need for food or sleep, frustrated tears were all I had.

I later realized that I was experiencing "pink cloud syndrome," a condition first described in the context of Alcoholics Anonymous (AA), in people recovering from alcohol use disorders. Others call it the honeymoon phase of recovery. In the first stages of recovery, recovering addicts feel a sense of exhilaration and euphoria, a high that almost matches the effects of using drugs or alcohol. They are emboldened by sobriety. Pink cloud syndrome can last weeks, even months. In my case, it lasted the entire year I lived in Colorado; it was definitely there at the summit of Pikes Peak and at the finish line of the Colorado Marathon. Feeling optimistic and having a positive outlook can help with recovery, but it can also make you feel invincible—and the higher the high, the farther the fall. When the pink cloud fades, disappointment, dysphoria, and even relapse can ensue. When I moved back to New Jersey, my pink cloud went from solid bubblegum pink to wispy, shredded, half-eaten cotton candy.

To avoid relapse, I had to stay true to myself and avoid triggers. I stood in front of the fridge, which was full of food after a trip to the grocery store. The house was quiet and still felt unfamiliar after only a month of living there. The cool air and bright light of the fridge washed over me as I searched for something to eat. Suddenly, I was gripped with panic as an overwhelming urge to binge took hold. The inner demon—the unwelcome voice I hadn't heard in ages—whispered in my ear, *Go ahead. It will make you feel better.* I had an excuse to give in. I was stressed out in a new place, lonely even though I no longer lived alone, and the idea of bingeing wrapped its arms around me like a comforting hug. I could bury my stress at the bottom of a pint of cookie dough ice cream. But would it make me feel better? To backslide when I had come so far? I slammed the fridge shut and raced upstairs to change into running clothes. Sneakers laced, I bolted out the door, as far away from temptation as my legs would carry me.

Every time I felt my resolve weakening, I put on my sneakers and ran. I ran. And I ran. And I ran some more. I pushed past the disruptive thoughts and left them in the dust. Beyond my driveway was a maze of quiet, narrow, tree-lined streets. They wound through nearby lake communities, far enough away from the major roads for me to not hear any traffic. There, I could run uninterrupted, looping together segments of roads that passed by private sandy beaches and lakeside houses, until I felt ready to go home. Sometimes I took my dog, Chief, with me. A feisty lab mix we'd rescued from South Carolina, he practically mauled me at the prospect of a walk or run every time I picked up his leash. When he joined me for short three-mile runs, he set a frenzied four-legged pace that left me gasping for breath as soon as we got out the door. Other times Rich came with me, challenging himself to try something new. He was a swimmer, not a runner. I was never sure if he loved running, or if he just loved me enough to stay by my side, but either way, he kept up.

Then I found other people to run with, this time on a soccer field. The adult recreational soccer league played weekly games on local grass and turf fields when they were not in use by youth leagues and high school teams, and it was designed for people like me: ex–high school athletes who still loved the sport. We might not be fast, but we had the muscle memory needed to shoot and take corner kicks. I excitedly pulled on shin guards, socks, and shiny new cleats as if I were getting dressed for the first day of school. I ran the length of the field, waiting for a chance to pass or shoot, watching the play and shouting to my teammates in a soccer dialect I hadn't spoken in years. Playing soccer again and using my body in a positive, active way reaffirmed my desire to be healthy; I just needed to stay the course.

I had never felt healthier or stronger than I did at the finish line of the Colorado Marathon. The pain of that first marathon was long forgotten; all I could remember was the glory of finishing the race. So why not run it again?

Rich, my mom, and I flew to Denver forty-eight hours before my second Colorado Marathon. Rich was ready for his first half-marathon, after months of training with me, and I was going to run the full. Having completed another twelve-week training plan, I felt confident. The day before the race, we walked around Boulder and then drove to Chautauqua Park, one of my favorite local hiking spots a few miles away. We labored up the first quarter mile of the trail. "This trail was much easier to hike when I lived in Denver," I told them, stopping to pick up a pinecone. The spines pricked my fingertips. "I made it all the way to the top of the Flatirons in no time." But now the Flatirons looked like skyscrapers, and I was breathless coming from sea level to 5,400 feet of elevation overnight. How was I going to run 26.2 miles if I was crippled by the altitude? There simply was not enough time to acclimatize. My confidence rolled back down the hill we had just climbed, and my lungs wanted to follow, back to thicker, oxygen-rich air.

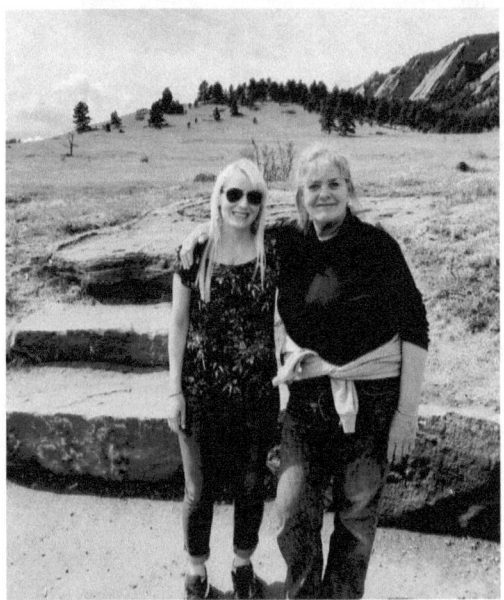

Hiking with my mom before the race

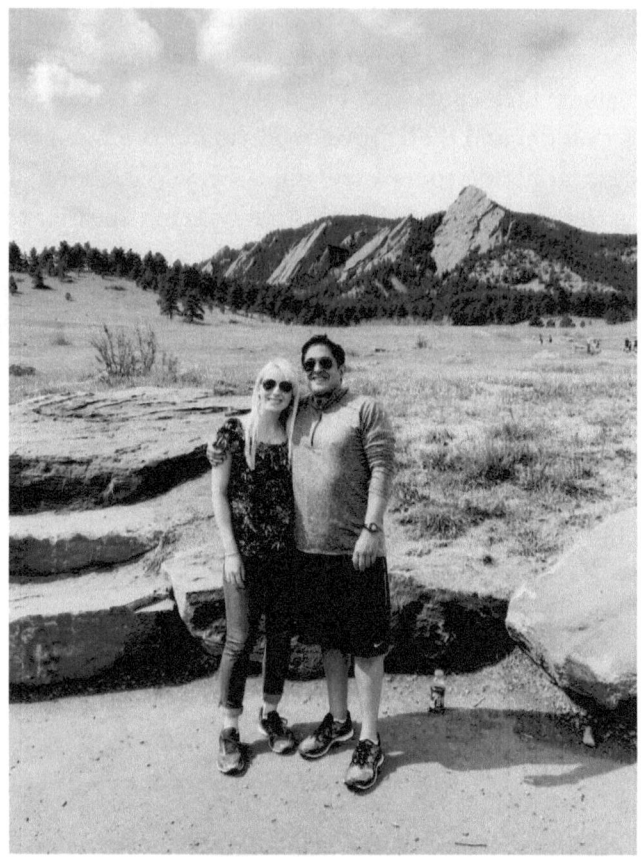

With Rich before the race

Nine minutes and thirty seconds per mile was a decent pace at the start of the race the next morning. But a pace that normally felt comfortable was now exhausting, and I was working a hundred times harder than usual to maintain it. I wondered how Rich was doing, farther down Poudre Canyon at the start of the half-marathon. "Wow! You just came from sea level to run a marathon in the Mile High City? That's amazing!" The runners next to me, gliding effortlessly along, were obviously Coloradan and recognized how foolish my attempt was. As the miles wore on and the temperature warmed, my pace slowed and I started to worry. How long could I keep this up?

At mile 21, I was past "the wall" and into the final stretch of the race. My mom and Rich waited on a grassy knoll beside the road, shaded from the sun, ready to spur me on with words of encouragement. The fact that Rich had already finished his half-marathon was a reminder of how long my feet had been relentlessly striking the ground. I was fatigued and weary. My lips were dry, and I felt thirsty, signs of dehydration. I hadn't been drinking enough, and it was too late to catch up. On the twenty-third mile, I crossed a hot, dry field, and a wave of light-headedness hit me. I went from upright, to hunched, to splayed out in the grass. My race was over.

I crawled off the course toward the air-conditioned car. "Good job, Cait," my mom said. "You gave it your all." She handed me a big bottle of water. I was crushed: It was my first DNF. DID NOT FINISH. For long-distance runners, a DNF is a rejection, a mark of failure. It puts your name at the bottom of the results list, so far down that it is almost as if you weren't there on race day. There is no consolation prize for finishing 23 miles, or even 26, when the goal is 26.2. Those three letters were as caustic to my ego as the bold F on my first medical school exam.

My gut reaction was to wallow in self-pity and shame myself for failing. *You're not good enough. You're not a REAL runner. You could have tried harder.* Shame takes shallow cuts and turns them into deep scars; it turns minor disappointments into catastrophic failures and turns you against yourself. *Not only are you a bad runner, you're a bad person.* This fucked-up way of thinking was familiar to me. It was the same negative self-talk that had invaded my mind when I looked in the mirror and saw "fat" no matter how much weight I had lost, the same self-talk that told me I was disgusting and unlovable when I stuck my finger in my throat. But in truth, it was one bad day, one small speed bump on a long road. DNF did not mean that I was not a good runner.

If you can push past shame, failure can be one of the greatest motivators for the human brain. Falling just short of a goal is in some ways even more motivating than actually achieving it. Dopamine is released in our brains in *anticipation* of a reward. If we don't reach the reward but there is a chance we can reach it next time, then we will continue to pursue that reward. This works best with short-term rewards, or quick fixes that make the limbic system happy, like scratch-off lottery tickets or playing Candy Crush. But pursuing a long-term goal and delaying gratification—such as reaching the finish line of a marathon—also increases dopamine. It strengthens the relationship between the limbic system and the prefrontal cortex. *I worked hard to achieve this; remember how good this felt and remind me to do it again.* Rather than working against each other, these parts of the brain team up, and the result is resilience and the ability to press on in the face of failure. That meant this DNF would not be my last attempt at a marathon.

That evening, we drove north to the Stanley Hotel, an iconic white building with a brick-red roof that stood out boldly against the backdrop of the mountains. The Stanley, featured in Stephen King's *The Shining*, was over one hundred years old, with an elegance and historic charm unmatched by any other hotel in Estes Park. The town was still quiet in May, before the snow melted off the trails and the onslaught of summer travelers arrived to hike them. We sat on the front porch, sinking into white wicker chairs and sipping Redrum Punch (a nod to the movie) while we waited for a table in the dining room. The view was spectacular, with the jagged peaks of the Rocky Mountains capped in snow in the distance.

12 | PERFECT MATCH

"Walk with me," Rich said, reaching for my hand. Ripples of pain moved up my legs with each step down the staircase to the gardens below. The downhill part of the race had destroyed my quads. We walked slowly among the flower beds and into the perfectly trimmed juniper hedge maze, gazing out at the mountains in the distance. It looked more like a movie set or painting than real life. "I'm so proud of you for finishing your first half-marathon," I told him. "I can't do what you do," he replied. "I don't know how you run 26 miles. You're a great runner, Cait. Don't let this get you down." He was right. I had to break away from the black-and-white thinking that dictated my life. I could still be a good runner without finishing the marathon, the same way I could be a good student without being the valedictorian; I could be good at a lot of things without being perfect at them. If there was anything I had learned from anorexia, it was that perfection was unattainable.

Rich knelt to the ground and pulled out a diamond ring from his pocket. He told me how much he loved me. "I was planning on giving this to you at the finish line of the marathon. Will you marry me?" If I had known a proposal was waiting for me at the finish line, maybe I would have pushed through the dizziness and dehydration. Maybe it would have been the motivation I needed. But it didn't matter—I had found my perfect match, and he was proposing to me in the perfect place. Colorado would always have a piece of my heart, but I had found my new home, and it was not confined to a location. My home was Rich, the person who saw the darkness and light within me and loved me for both. He turned a bad day into the best day, failure was forgotten, and together we watched the sun set over the Rockies.

Chapter 13

RUNNING FROM PERFECTION

"Eye of the Tiger" blared from the speakers at the start line of the Philadelphia Marathon, just yards away from the famous *Rocky* steps, and the first group of elite runners took off at full stride. Several corrals behind and hundreds of feet away, I waited for my chance to move forward and start the clock for my third marathon. The view of the city was inspiring in the early morning, with flags from dozens of countries lining Benjamin Franklin Parkway and the illuminated clock tower of Philadelphia City Hall directly ahead. The jittery energy of ten thousand runners lined up shoulder to shoulder and loud music pumping from the speakers galvanized the atmosphere. I waited impatiently in the chilly air, stretching my calves and hopping lightly on my feet to stay limber and warm. I balled my fists with anticipation, warming my fingertips.

Failure had fueled the desire to succeed, to reach the finish line again. By the time the Philadelphia Marathon arrived in late November, six months after my failed attempt in Colorado, I was eager for redemption. The marathon traditionally took place the weekend before Thanksgiving, which meant it was usually a cool, crisp fall day—perfect for running. Fifty degrees Fahrenheit is an ideal temperature for a marathon, the temperature at which a runner's body performs the best, and my body was no exception. Having regained weight and health, I no longer wore layers of sweaters and huddled near heating vents to stay warm. Now I thrived in the cold and withered in the heat.

After a few miles of warming up, most runners shed layers and tossed their gloves and windbreakers onto the street, draping the curbs with the most expensive piles of litter the city had ever seen. Colorful North Face, Nike, and Brooks apparel lay next to shriveled cigarette butts and food wrappers. I chose to run in shorts and a T-shirt. This time I was prepared with energy gels and a hydration vest, a purchase I had made after the Colorado marathon desiccated me from a grape into a raisin. I never wanted to feel thirsty during a race again.

The Philadelphia Marathon is a mostly flat race that started at Eakins Oval, the traffic circle near the Philadelphia Museum of Art. The course wove through neighborhoods I was familiar with—Center City, Old City, West Philly—and then along the Schuylkill River to Manayunk, before looping back toward the art museum for the final six miles of the race.

Familiarity was a double-edged sword. Before I signed up for the race, I was hesitant to return to Philly to run, because even though it was only miles from my new home in New Jersey, the ghosts of my past lived within the city limits. My brain associated Philly with my most self-destructive habits. While there were good memories—going to restaurants and museums with my friends and family, barhopping with co-residents, walking through city parks with Rich—there were also awful memories of specific places where I had made bad choices.

My old apartment was the site of ravenous binges, and certain bars in Center City triggered memories of too many tequila shots, dancing and making out with strangers, and feeling out of control. Those places were crime scenes in my mind, and I did not want to revisit them. How would I feel running past them? Would my ghosts come out to haunt me and sabotage my race, filling my mind with bad memories on replay for 26 miles? I wasn't sure I could handle that. But there was only one way to find out.

I took off, racing down Arch Street through Chinatown. The building on the corner of Ninth Street was a converted warehouse, full of spacious one- and two-bedroom apartments with modern amenities. My apartment had been on the eighth floor, above the noise of the city streets. I remembered the high ceilings, the wildlife artwork that hung on the walls, the big purple area rug, the huge windows that let sunlight in. It was the first place that felt luxurious and safe, much nicer than the studio apartment on Walnut Street where the rats outnumbered the tenants. I pushed down the negative thoughts associated with it—the sad and lonely nights spent binge eating on the granite countertops or barely finishing a bowl of soup when I was too depressed to eat—and focused only on the positive. Positive thoughts seemed to energize my body and make me run faster, and that felt good.

Whenever I passed a place that evoked bad memories, I kicked up my pace a bit and replaced emotion with physical exertion, weakness with strength. I ran from the ghosts, just as I had during my first half-marathon in medical school. Like the fans who lined the streets, they motivated me to run harder. When I passed places like Washington Square Park, where Rich and I had walked hand in hand after a romantic dinner, I let waves of good memories and nostalgia wash over me. Mile after mile, I revisited my former life in Philadelphia and rewrote the script. I turned every block, every street corner into something positive, forming new memories that would merge with the triumph of finishing another marathon.

"You can do it, Caitlin!" "Great job! Keep going!" Excited fans, who cared enough to read my name on the front of my bib, shouted words of encouragement directed right at me. The entire city buzzed with the energy of the race, with droves of fans cheering, ringing cowbells, and holding up huge signs with running puns: "Chafing the dream!" "26.2 . . . because 26.3 would be crazy!" "The rats don't run this city—you do!" They offered tissues, snacks, and bottles of water to any runner who needed them. On marathon day, the City of Brotherly Love earned its nickname, with so many city dwellers taking part from the sidelines.

I hit the halfway point of the race feeling strong and headed out on Kelly Drive, an out-and-back section that covered the last 12 miles of the course along the Schuylkill River. I was pummeled by the wind and the rolling hills leading to the neighborhood of Manayunk, where the crowds were even rowdier and more excited to see the runners. Instead of handing out water, they proffered cups of beer and shots of liquor like it was a Mardi Gras celebration. Confetti—and our sneakers—stuck to the sticky, beer-slicked pavement. As I hit mile 21, the familiar pain of hitting the wall and then running through it settled into my quads and calves.

Before the race, Rich had asked, "Does running a marathon get easier every time you do it? Is it less painful?" "No, it hurts like hell every time," I said. "The difference is knowing to expect it." But it was more than expecting pain; it was *accepting* it. Leaning into the pain and embracing it, taking the last leg of the journey side by side with it like a fellow soldier marching into battle. And so I dug in, carrying the pain with me. Pain was transient, an obligatory part of a marathon that would only make me stronger at the finish. I paused at the flag marking the start of mile 24 and thought, *This is where your legs stop working and your mind pushes you the rest of the way.* I finished the race in four hours and thirty-one minutes, cutting five minutes off my first marathon time. I was nowhere near the front of the pack, but I felt victorious.

After my second successful marathon, it was easy to imagine running another, and then another. Between training for half- and full marathon races, running longer distances became my new normal. When I laced up my sneakers, my body expected a long run, like a sled dog ready to hit the tundra as soon as its harness was in place. Three miles, a number I used to stop at on the treadmill, was now my warm-up. As I built up mileage before each race, my base level of fitness continued to improve, and waking up to run 10 or 12 miles became easier. I wondered how much distance my legs could cover if my mind was 100 percent committed to it. What would happen if I ran a marathon distance, and then I kept going? Would there be fuel left in the tank?

Running was a habit, a healthy one, a replacement for the destructive habits that had taken up so much of my focus. Instead of draining my energy the way bulimia had, running replenished it. On some level I knew that fact when I started running in medical school and residency, but it didn't stick until I became a marathoner. My brain obviously liked to form habits, but it didn't discriminate between good and bad; I had to choose, and I could choose to run.

While I pounded the pavement for hours at a time, my mind was free to wander. Other questions about running bubbled up in my thoughts. What defines success as a runner? Is it finishing every race, finishing it in a certain time, beating the competition, or besting your own personal record? As a goal-oriented person, I liked the idea of reaching a finishing line and vying to get faster with each successive race, but I would never be fast by any standard. Nine-minute miles are not competitive at any distance. My high school was so small that it did not have a track, and I was not coached from an early age like the athletes who end up in the Olympics. I would never run a five-minute mile or win a race, and that was fine. I didn't care about beating the person next to me either; I was competing against myself, for myself.

But what I really wanted was to not care about any of it. I wanted to throw out all the metrics, like I had thrown away the scale when I moved to Colorado. For too long, I had used arbitrary numbers to validate my self-worth—the number on the scale, the number of calories I ate, the numeric size on clothing labels—and I was fucking tired of it. Even the treadmill gave me useless, irritating feedback, with its glaring red digital display measuring how far I ran or how many calories I burned, as if those things were what defined a good runner.

I wanted to run for the pure joy of it, to feel my body move freely and powerfully without worrying about how fast or how far I was going. I wanted to defy the rules I had set for myself and refute the need to be perfect at everything I did. The next time I went for a run, I left my Garmin watch at home and let the miles pass by at whatever pace felt good for my muscles. I measured my success as a runner by the way I felt while I was running, rather than any split time or pace. I ran from perfection.

"How was your run?" Rich asked, as I pulled off my hydration pack and gloves in the doorway to our kitchen. Cheeks flushed and slightly windburned from the frosty winter air, I told him it was great. "What was your time?" he asked. "I have no idea," I said, beaming. Running without rules or expectations made me happy.

13 | RUNNING FROM PERFECTION

Once I freed myself from perfection and its arbitrary metrics, I could feel *profoundly* the benefits of running on my mind and body. It was not merely a mental distraction; it was meditation, therapy, and art expressed through physical movement. To call it a habit was selling it short. Running was the most effective therapy I had ever tried, and the cheapest. The only cost was the price of a pair of sneakers. And the results were reliable and reproducible.

After the first few miles of a run, my mind became focused on the act of running itself, and nothing else mattered. I paid attention to the movements of my body, noticing the rhythm of my steps and the elegance of my stride. The longer I ran, the more I noticed each muscle group engaging in my quads, my calves, and my core. I matched the cadence of my steps to the inhale and exhale of each breath. I was present in the moment, removed from the anxiety and tension of everyday life. My body was a powerful machine, and my mind was at ease. Even my dog, Chief, could sense a change in my energy and mood. Instead of bounding ahead, he ran by my side and looked up at me expectantly, waiting for my next move. My composure was contagious.

Ironically, the less I cared about numbers, the better an athlete I became. I found myself reaching for a greater challenge, something bigger than a marathon, something that would test my mental fortitude and the love of running in its purest form.

Danielle, who had taken me on my first trail run in Red Rocks Park, gave me an idea. Being active and outdoors was an integral part of her life, and she was a natural athlete. She told me about her attempts at the Leadville Trail 100 Run, a punishing multiday ultramarathon based in Leadville, Colorado, with 18,000 feet of elevation change and rugged terrain that attracted the best trail runners every year. It was aptly nicknamed the

"Race Across the Sky," as it crossed several mountain passes and peaked at an altitude above 12,000 feet. I couldn't believe that anyone would willingly suffer through 100 miles of trail running, not to mention the sleep deprivation that came with spending several nights in the mountains. Although Danielle's first two attempts had been unsuccessful, she never gave up and ultimately conquered the race on her third try.

"You should run an ultramarathon with me!" she texted. Her enthusiasm was persuasive, even through text message and across two time zones. "If you like running and hiking, you'll love this." Before that, I had never heard of an ultramarathon. An ultramarathon is technically any race longer than the marathon distance of 26.2 miles. The most common distance is 50 kilometers, but races vary significantly in time and distance. Some cover a specified distance, such as 200 miles, and some last for a predetermined amount of time, such as twenty-four hours. Sometimes the winner is the one who covers the greatest distance within a time period, and other times the winner is the last person standing. Most ultras take place on trails with natural obstacles such as mud, hills, and rocky terrain, all of which—in addition to the distance—add to the effort of running.

Compared to marathons, which attract crowds of thousands of runners, ultramarathons draw much smaller numbers—sometimes hundreds, sometimes dozens, sometimes only handfuls of people. Only 0.03 percent of the US population runs ultras, partly because they require more endurance and self-support, but also because there are smaller rewards for winning. Winning a major marathon comes with acclaim and a cash prize, maybe a book deal or sponsorship; winning an ultramarathon earns you a finisher's medal and muddy, smelly shoes.

While ultramarathons are still niche in the sport of running, they are gaining popularity, with the growth rate over the past

13 | RUNNING FROM PERFECTION

ten to fifteen years exceeding that of marathons and 5K races. There has also been a rise in the number of women running ultras, with female runners now representing close to 25 percent of participants. Men have always been faster at shorter distances, but the longer the race, the closer women come to closing the gender gap, with women's paces nearly matching men's by the end of 100-mile events. Ultramarathons also attract "older" runners, people over the age of forty, whose fast-twitch muscle fibers for sprinting have been replaced by slow-twitch fibers for endurance.

I had to admit, I was intrigued. An ultramarathon sounded perfectly *un*-perfect. A challenge for marathoners who wanted to explore their love of running and defy the rules of road races, to run without the luxury of flat pavement beneath their feet. I envisioned running along dirt trails, then hiking up the steep parts, spatters of dirt and mud caking up the sides of my calves, and pain in places I was not used to from stumbling over rocks and tree roots. My pace would fluctuate up and down like the hills. My sneakers would be destroyed from the effort and would never wash clean again. My salty skin would need to be power washed from all the dirt and grit. I would get lost in nature, but hopefully just metaphorically. Was I crazy to think this sounded alluring? What drove other runners to the start lines of these intense, physically demanding races?

"Let's do it!" I texted back. I was about to find out just how much fuel I had in the tank and how my brain could keep me running, even on empty.

Chapter 14

TYPE II FUN

On November 5, 2022, it was humid and unseasonably hot in the Pine Barrens of New Jersey, as if the Jersey Devil himself were warming the woods with his fiery breath. I waited at the start of the Batona Trail Races dressed lightly in a moisture-wicking T-shirt and shorts, knowing I would be on the trail until the temperature rose to a high of 78°F by the afternoon. My muscles twitched in anticipation of the pain I would endure by the end of the race. This was my second ultramarathon, and I knew what to expect: I would feel ragged from heat and exertion, surf a wave of emotions during seven hours of running, take moments to enjoy the scenery, eat and drink constantly without ever feeling hungry or sated, and eventually come off the trail exhausted but content.

The Batona Trail is a sandy, mostly flat 53.5-mile trail through the pine forests in the southern part of New Jersey. One of the longest trails in the tiny state, it traverses the Brendan T. Byrne, Wharton, and Bass River State Forests as it heads southeast toward the Jersey Shore. My race spanned the last 33 miles of the trail, and it would be the farthest distance I had attempted so far.

Two years earlier, I had run my first ultramarathon, which took place in the rolling hills of California along the American River. Admittedly, I registered for the race without knowing what I was really signing up for. I was excited to run it with Danielle, and to take a break from the dreary, snowless winter in New Jersey. I daydreamed about running freely, arms spread wide, traversing 31.4 miles as effortlessly and gracefully as a deer prancing through the woods. But the reality was that it would kick my ass in more ways than one, and I would fly home to my husband hobbling with a bruised ego.

The Way Too Cool 50K was held in the town of Cool, California, which, apropos of its name, had the relaxed vibe of a small mountain town and was rife with trendy coffee shops and restaurants. The course was scenic, mostly single-track trail that traced the curve of the American River and followed sections of the Western States Trail, with a total vertical elevation change of 4,800 feet. For a March race, I had expected the cool temperatures and sunny skies that come with spring in California, but for race day, freezing rain was forecast. The residents of Cool were thrilled, commenting on the drought and the need for rain. I warily sipped my caramel latte in a coffeehouse next to Danielle. "I can't wait for the rain," the barista said. "Perfect day to sit on the couch and watch movies all day." *Or run an ultramarathon,* I thought, pitying myself. Somehow, the rain clouds that seemed to follow me on long training runs in New Jersey had made it all the way to the West Coast.

On race day, the sky was shrouded in bloated gray clouds that held the impending rain like expanding water balloons about to burst. Teeth chattering, I warmed up by stretching and walking along the gravel road leading up to the start line. As the first few race miles ticked slowly by, I could feel my body temperature start to rise with the effort of running. I was using far more energy in navigating twists and turns, uneven surfaces, and exposed tree roots than I ever had in a road race. Roads were linear and predictable; trails were anything but. In all my long-distance training, I had neglected to think about how training runs on pavement would translate to the trail.

I anxiously called out to Danielle ahead of me, "I don't think I'm built for this!" She laughed and kept moving, knowing that I had no choice but to finish what I had started. She told me it was okay to take walking breaks, especially uphill; I heeded her advice, even though it contradicted everything I had learned in road marathons. Marathons call for constant running and speed. But ultramarathons encourage breaks to eat, drink, walk up hills, chat with aid station crews, offer a hand if someone falls, even cry your eyes out—whatever feels right in the moment.

Halfway through the race, the freezing rain commenced. It would not stop again until I left the town of Cool. At first, it was fun splashing through ankle-deep puddles and letting the raindrops bounce off my skin, washing the sweat away. But then the rain seeped into every fiber of my clothing, and the constant sloshing, squishing, and dripping became its own sloppy, wet melody. Feelings of self-doubt crept in like the icy chill of the rain, and that made the landscape look more dramatic and difficult: bigger puddles, steeper hills, sagging tree branches reaching down like tired old arms.

When I could no longer feel my fingers and my skin had chafed raw, I wanted to stop. Tears welled up in my eyes and spilled over, but blending into the beads of rain streaming down my face, they were invisible to anyone around me. Would willpower be enough to get me through the race? The idea of quitting, and the promise of a scalding hot shower and dry clothes, was enticing. But I kept moving.

"Welcome to Goat Hill!" a man boomed, handing out strands

of red licorice to the runners as they started the steep ascent from mile 25 to mile 26. Bearded and a bit unkempt, the elderly man was a local whose annual tradition was to cheer the runners on at the crux of the race. He was the only person on the sidelines between aid stations. The climb seemed too steep for human feet and more fitting for a mountain goat's hooves. It turned my run into a grueling hike, and I pitched forward so far that my fingertips brushed the muddy earth. It was *too* hard, and the desire to quit resurfaced. At the top of Goat Hill, I told the support crew at the aid station that I was finished and asked how I could get off the course. I had done enough. Who could fault me for not finishing, when I had already run a marathon distance on a rugged trail? "Well, just keep going another 5.4 miles to the finish line and then you'll be off the course. There's no way out here." It was a slap to my ruddy, frozen cheek.

Danielle sidled up to me. "Every step you take past a marathon distance will be the farthest you've ever run. You can do this." She asked me what I needed to finish the race, offering energy gels, snacks, and the freedom to cry as many tears as I wanted. It was enough to make me laugh, take a deep breath, and follow her lead back onto the trail. Even this far along, Danielle was hopping along the trail like a hare, at home in the forest. Her stride was relaxed and effortless. Inspired by her stamina and agility, I picked my feet up a bit higher and dug into the last muddy stretch of trail.

Just one more step, just one more step became the desperate mantra I repeated in my mind. One step became ten, then one hundred, and then I lost count, focused on placing one foot in front of the other. I finished the race by Danielle's side, exactly seven hours after we had started. As we walked back to the car, the rain poured down even harder, a punch line to the cruel joke nature had played on us. I was proud of myself for finishing when I had nearly given up. I was bent but not broken, with blistered

14 | TYPE II FUN

feet, swollen thighs, and a finisher's pint glass as proof of what my body had been through. It was a testament to the strength of my mind and its ability to command my body to keep going when I wanted to stop. Now that I had finished an ultramarathon, I could hang up the reins and never do one again.

As quickly as my mind forgot the pain of running a marathon, it forgot the pain of running an ultramarathon. All I could remember was the feeling of accomplishment at the end of the race. It was Type II fun. The Fun Scale, invented by rock climbers in the 1980s, is used by outdoor athletes to describe the type of enjoyment gained from adventures and misadventures. Type I fun is obvious, easy fun, like drinking margaritas, lying on the beach, or having dinner with friends. Type III fun, on the opposite end of the spectrum, is not fun at all: getting lost in the woods, missing a flight, a breakup—things you never want to do again. In the middle is Type II fun, which is often considered the most rewarding kind of fun.

Type II fun is hard, challenging, and uncomfortable while you are doing it, but you feel invigorated and alive afterward: trekking to Everest base camp, riding your bike across the country, or in my case, running an ultramarathon. With time, your memory phases out the miserable moments, and all you remember is the joy of it. Your brain interprets pain, like pleasure, as a stepping-stone to a long-awaited reward, and delaying a reward strengthens the prefrontal cortex. "Remember those huge blisters on my calves and ankles?" "Remember that giant knee-deep puddle and how we ran straight through it?" Months later, Danielle and I recalled how much fun we'd had.

My brain learned to associate trail running with feeling powerful, and that was vindication for my former self, the anorexic girl who was too weak to run a mile and then the bulimic girl who treated her body like a punching bag. I wanted to do it again, to have more Type II fun. I was grateful to have my health back, a second chance to be an athlete. That's how I found myself at the starting line of the Batona Trail Races—that and two years of working in healthcare during the COVID-19 pandemic. For hospital workers, emotional well-being and quality of life had taken a nosedive, as had the opportunity for travel and fitness. Organized races were nonexistent, and runners were encouraged to do virtual races instead; I wondered if the Philadelphia Marathon, with close to ten thousand runners, would ever safely return. I wore my surgical mask for ten hours a day at work, taking shallow, stifled breaths and adjusting it on my face constantly. I forgot what my co-workers' faces looked like.

After work, alone, I shed the mask and went running around my neighborhood, sucking in deep, luxurious breaths of fresh air to expand my lungs. Being free from the chaos and constraints that existed within the hospital walls heightened the experience of running outdoors. When the pandemic waned, I signed up for the first trail race I could find. Ultramarathons, with only a few hundred people and plenty of space between runners, were back in action.

In the months leading up to the Batona race, I bought trail running shoes and trained on dirt trails—things I should have done the first time. I focused on my nutrition before, during, and after runs. This time, I would be physically prepared so I would not have to rely solely on mental stamina. During the Way Too Cool 50K, I had become aware of the strong connection between emotional state and physical performance. Seven hours on my feet was a lot of time to think and to study the way mood affected my running. Negative thinking—*You're too fat, you're not pretty enough, you could lose a few pounds*—was the gateway to anorexia, to low self-esteem and shame. As a runner, negative thinking was a guaranteed way to fail. *You're too slow. You'll never make it up this hill.* When I talked down to myself and doubted my ability to keep going, it manifested physically as hunched shoulders, slumped posture, clumsy steps, and fatigue. It convinced me to slow to a walk or stop completely.

Positivity was the only option; I had to block out intrusive thoughts the same way I blocked out urges to binge. I had to run with my head held high, looking straight ahead instead of down at my feet. I had to focus on positive thoughts during my training runs, and run to positive, upbeat music. The better my mood, the stronger my gait. Instead of praying to the running gods to allow me to take one more step, I found a mantra, a few simple words to motivate me and turn my mood around during a trail race. *Powerful. Perseverance.* Those words were a reminder of the hard things I had endured—my eating disorder, medical school, residency, poverty—and a reminder that I was strong enough to get through any obstacle in front of me.

On the morning of the Batona Trail race, Rich dropped me off at the starting area, where a few dozen runners were shaking out their limbs and counting energy gels and snacks before tucking them into hydration vests. I was running alone, without Danielle, and I would have to motivate myself. I stretched next to a few lean, athletic women; I had no doubt they would leave me in the dust. But there were no sideways glances to assess me as a competitor; they introduced themselves, and we chatted about running.

The ultrarunning community was friendly, encouraging, and humble. Ego was not as important as it was at a marathon start line, where runners wanted to qualify for other races or win prize money. The only prize here was the intrinsic reward that came with finishing the challenge. Huddled at the start, we were like a herd of caribou about to trek across a frozen tundra; it felt like a migration, a pilgrimage, rather than a race. We would start the journey as a group, and we would endure it as a group. No one wanted to declare themselves a front-runner. The race director blew the whistle, and then we were off.

The race quickly veered off the road onto single-track trail lined by conifers. The trail was carpeted with freshly fallen pine needles, which scented the air and made the surface slippery. Each stride was springy, as if I were running on pillows instead of soft sandy soil and pine needles. While my joints were grateful for the cushioning, my brain could not figure out how forcefully my feet were striking the ground. Each carefully placed step required a little extra effort to stay balanced.

At the first aid station, six miles in, I felt good. With the aid station crew cheering me onward, I continued along the trail, at times stopping to take pictures of the sun streaming through the forest. If life is a journey, not a destination, the same could be said of trail racing. Crossing the finish line was a single moment in time. The things that would be etched into memory, consolidated by the emotional experience of running an ultra, were the sights and sounds of the forest, the calm and peace of being surrounded by nature. The race itself faded into the background as I focused on the sound of my breathing and the smell of pine. It was meditative and reminded me of hiking in the Rocky Mountains.

I was feeling overwhelmingly positive halfway through the race when the valve on my hydration pack broke. My precious water spilled out like a geyser, and the sandy soil greedily consumed it. Miles away from the next aid station, I had no water, and the temperature was rising steadily. Everything around me screamed for water—the crunchy pine needles beneath my feet, the low-lying plants that extended their dry fingerlike branches to scratch my exposed thighs as I scurried along the trail. My mouth immediately felt dry, and I feared another DNF.

14 | TYPE II FUN

I was overheating like an old car on a lone stretch of desert highway. I hated running in the heat; it was when I felt the weakest as a runner. I had to keep my energy up somehow, so I pulled an energy gel from my vest. Cherry Lime GU stuck to the roof of my mouth like glue. There was nothing to wash it down with, but I knew I had to swallow the paste that tasted like children's cold medicine. Energy gels were packed with easily digestible carbohydrates, which I needed as much as water if I was going to finish the race.

When I was anorexic, I ate as few calories as I could each day. I dreaded dense foods like energy gels, packed with 200 calories in a single sticky mouthful. But as an ultramarathoner, they were an essential part of my race. If I wanted to run that far, I had to consume 200 to 300 calories per hour, stopping at aid stations for chips, peanut butter and jelly sandwiches, pickles, gummy bears—anything I could find to keep me going.

Beyond mile 20, my pace slowed to a crawl, but surprisingly, no one passed me. Every member of the running herd was just as fatigued and overheated as I was. The familiar aches and pains settled into my hips, knees, and ankles. Everything felt stiff and sore, but oddly, it felt better to keep running than to walk or rest. When I reached the aid station at mile 22 and refilled my pack, I knew nothing would stop me from finishing the race. *Powerful. Perseverance.* Those were the only thoughts I allowed myself for the rest of the race. I stomped them into the ground with each determined step forward.

"Which way is the Batona Trail?" I asked. "I'm 32 miles into this race, and I'd like to be done!" I was on the last mile; the trail crossed over a paved road and then disappeared. Somehow I had ended up lost, running into the middle of a campsite where a group of Boy Scouts and their leader were making a campfire. They looked at me, a disheveled blonde Yeti who had emerged from the woods and was lumbering toward them. I was sweaty, dirty, and contorting myself to stretch my right leg as my calf cramped up. The scout leader pointed me back toward the trail, thankfully only a hundred feet away. The race had almost turned into Type III fun: lost in the woods. The wide-eyed stares from the scouts told me I was doing something incredible, that they were impressed. In that moment, I was impressed too. Years of running had transformed me from sick to healthy and into a real athlete again.

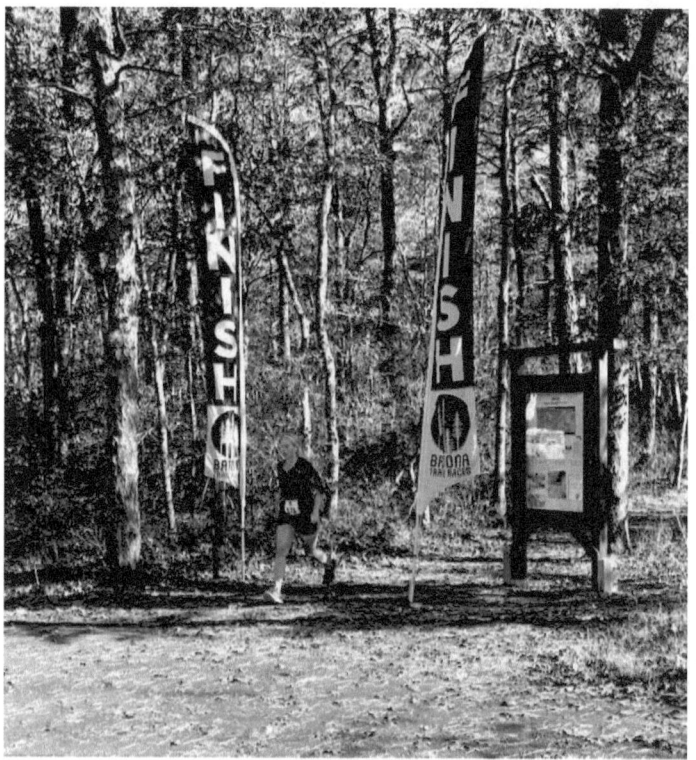

Batona Trail Races finish line

14 | TYPE II FUN

I sprinted the last tenth of a mile, determined to finish strong. At least, it felt like sprinting; maybe I could have beaten glacial flow. Six hours and forty-five minutes—faster than my first 50-kilometer race. Across the finish line, Rich waited to give me a big hug. He was my husband now, and he wanted to take care of me. "I'll take you out for anything you want: eggs, blueberry pancakes, pizza, ice cream, cake . . ." he said. As he rambled off a decadent post-race menu, I loved him even more. Food was no longer the enemy, and I was starving.

Chapter 15

EXERCISE JUNKIE

Food was my first drug, but it was not my last. Food is a reward, stimulating dopamine release in the brain and activating the opioid system, which plays an important role in the regulation of food intake and hedonic overeating. Sometimes eating is driven by physical hunger, and other times it is driven by reward hunger—the desire to eat as an answer to stress or boredom, or as a way to celebrate. With reward hunger, food choices are driven by emotion and provide comfort rather than nutrients. That is why emotional eating is more likely to push us past the point of fullness. Highly palatable foods, rich in sugar and fat, are the most calorie-dense, filling foods, and they are also the biggest triggers for the opioid system. Far more dangerous than donuts and cake are compounds that activate opioid receptors, such as heroin, morphine, and fentanyl. It is not hard to see how the mind of someone with an eating disorder, especially binge eating, can mimic that of a drug addict.

But there is another powerful habit that stimulates opioid receptors, one that is seemingly healthier than binge eating or abusing a substance: exercise. Habitual exercise can become a cross-addiction, a way to substitute one reward for another. For some people, like me, exercise can be the key to recovery from an eating disorder; for others, it can be a gateway drug.

From Athlete to Eating Disorder

According to a 2018 report from the *Journal of Clinical Sport Psychology*, up to 45 percent of female athletes and 19 percent of male athletes experience an eating disorder; and among female athletes, the risk of developing an eating disorder is twice as high in adolescents as it is in adults.[21] These statistics are not surprising. As we have discussed, the adolescent brain is more vulnerable to bad habits, addictions, and societal pressures. During adolescence, we develop norms related to body image and health practices based on what we learn from parents, coaches, mentors, and peers. We also absorb content from social media and ads that promote enhanced and unrealistic body images, and those ideals seep into our subconscious definition of beauty. In a 2015 study of undergraduate students, females were 3.5 times more likely than males to follow at least one type of health and fitness-related social media account, and 2.4 times more likely to have an eating disorder if they "liked" or "followed" those accounts.[22] These numbers have increased in parallel with the rising use of multiple social media platforms among young adults. According to a 2024 report in *Eating Behaviors*, it is the type of content, rather than the time spent on social media, that has a negative impact on body image and eating behaviors, particularly when it comes to image-based platforms such as Snapchat.[23]

Competitive athletes are driven by the need to have the perfect body—or at least the perfect body for their sport—to excel. Sports that focus on the individual, such as track, gymnastics, dance, and ice skating, put all the performance demands on one person, leading to an overwhelming amount of stress and unrealistically high self-expectations. For wrestlers, this means being weighed in front of your team and excluded from competition if your weight is above the upper limit for that class. For ballet dancers and gymnasts, the aesthetic performance—looking lithe in a leotard—is as important as the athletic one. For runners, there is a belief that lower body weight and a lean physique will make you faster. If the winner of the 400-meter sprint is the skinniest girl on the team, and you want to win, then the answer must be that you need to lose weight.

In young athletes, a perfectionist attitude and desire to be the best is a double-edged sword, often encouraged by the people judging their performance, such as coaches, parents, and college recruiters. In the pursuit of the perfect athletic body, food and weight can become negatively associated with fitness, and this can incite a dangerous rigidity and self-discipline with respect to nutrition. This pattern can lead to disordered eating, and in turn, an eating disorder. Athletes at the highest levels of competition, and those who were indoctrinated into their sport at an early age, such as elite track runners who go on to compete in the Olympics, have the highest risk of developing these problems.

Disordered eating comes from a distorted relationship with food or with body image, and manifests as a spectrum of patterns and behaviors that do not fully meet the DSM-5 criteria for an eating disorder. Because the symptoms do not fit the textbook definition, disordered eating is often unrecognized, but it can be serious. Some practices include frequently weighing oneself, following diets or cleanses, skipping meals, and using diet pills or laxatives. For athletes, excessive exercise and fasting are often used as compensation for eating. Disordered eating can also mean avoiding food in social situations or cutting out food groups entirely. While disordered eating is thought to stem from conscious control of behaviors, it is not hard to imagine these behaviors turning into unconscious habits and uncontrollable obsessions that occupy one's thoughts every waking hour. In fact, it has been proposed that disordered eating may be related to OCD.[24]

The best example of disordered eating is orthorexia, an obsessive focus on "healthy" eating. People with orthorexia follow an inflexible set of self-imposed restrictions on diet with the goal of getting healthier or preventing disease. They truly believe they are doing something good for their health by eliminating unhealthy foods and performing purifying cleanses. Losing weight, intended or unintended, is a bonus. They spend most of their time choosing and preparing healthy food, and catastrophizing and feeling guilty when they cannot access "clean" food, to a degree that impairs daily functioning and mimics the obsessions and rituals seen in OCD. Orthorexia symptoms are quite common in people with anorexia and bulimia, and interestingly, more common in doctors and dieticians than in the general population.[25] Too much knowledge can be dangerous.

While males with disordered eating tend to be focused on gaining muscle mass, females are more focused on weight loss. For young female athletes, taking in inadequate calories while working toward higher levels of competition can lead to a severe energy imbalance. Previously known as the "female athlete triad," relative energy deficiency in sport, or RED-S, is a state of impaired physiological functioning due to low energy availability, which results in many intertwined problems: amenorrhea (lack of a menstrual period) in females, impaired metabolism, decreased bone mineral density (osteoporosis or osteopenia), and decreased immune function. Low energy availability may be intentional, as in the case of restricted or disordered eating, or it may be the result of exercise and energy expenditure that exceeds normal caloric intake.

Often, young female athletes lack the knowledge needed to

make good decisions about nutrition and how to properly fuel their bodies, and they rely on whatever their parents buy at the grocery store or copy their teammates' or friends' eating habits at school. This can leave them with a huge energy deficit that impairs athletic performance. The hormonal changes that accompany menstrual dysfunction, such as low estrogen, can have long-lasting effects on development, fertility, and bone health into adulthood. RED-S, like anorexia, is more common in sports that emphasize low body weight, such as running and gymnastics, but it is not exclusive to female athletes; males who compete in weight-class sports such as horse racing, weightlifting, and wrestling are also susceptible.

All these conditions are red flags for an impending eating disorder. Athletes at risk are often socially isolated, frequently injured with stress fractures and muscle strains, and preoccupied with food. They continue to train despite illness, injury, low energy levels, and overwhelming fatigue.

Sadly, despite behavioral signs and physical manifestations, eating disorders often go unnoticed or, worse, ignored. There are several screening inventories and questionnaires that have been developed to identify athletes at risk, such as the Eating Attitudes Test (EAT-26), the Brief Eating Disorder in Athletes Questionnaire (BEDA-Q), and the Athletic Milieu Direct Questionnaire (ADMQ), with strong evidence to support their use. The National Eating Disorders Association (NEDA) also offers an accessible online screening tool,[26] the data from which has been used in studies comparing athlete versus non-athlete participants.[27]

But how often are these tools implemented in everyday practice? Who is asking these questions of young female athletes? In a 2014 study of 123 high school coaches, 83 percent said they were comfortable talking about disordered eating with their athletes, yet only 40 percent reported having asked questions about their eating patterns. Only 24 percent of coaches had heard of the female athlete triad or RED-S, and 69 percent did not know that lack of periods could be related to bone loss and fractures.[28] Lack of awareness of symptoms is an ongoing issue, as evidenced by a 2022 study in *BMJ Open Sport & Exercise Medicine* that reported coaches surveyed were no more likely to identify symptoms than non-coach participants.[29] The coaches who were able to identify symptoms scored higher on mental health literacy tests and were more likely to recommend professional treatment once an eating disorder was identified. This highlights an opportunity to improve mental health literacy not only among coaches, but also among school nurses, guidance counselors, and, of course, parents.

When I was picked for the varsity soccer team, it was based on my ability to dribble and pass a ball and how quickly I could sprint a set distance during timed intervals. I was healthy to start, but as my performance deteriorated with the progression of my eating disorder, there was no check-in from my coach or a dietician to assess my eating habits or mental well-being. No one asked me if I missed my period, or if I was struggling to get through drills. No one asked me if soccer was driving my weight loss, or if something else was. As long as I showed up for practice, I was a part of the team. If I had been benched or sent to counseling, I would have rebelled against it, but it would have been an impactful lesson for the female athletes around me.

From Eating Disorder to Athlete

Hiking to alpine lakes, running marathons and ultramarathons, summitting Colorado fourteeners and Washington volcanoes. My brain interpreted all these physical activities as rewarding, but in a less obvious way than binge eating. I was getting my fix another way, through exercise, but because I had to work harder to get to the finish line or summit, the reward was longer-lasting and more meaningful.

As I said before, sports did not trigger my eating disorder. Just the opposite, they healed me. And I am not the only ultrarunner who has recovered from an eating disorder. Endurance sports attract survivors—people who have battled with eating disorders, abuse, drug and alcohol addiction, chronic illness, traumatic life events, and PTSD. While some people turn to religion or therapy groups for guidance, others find spirituality in the mountains or in long-distance running, swimming, cycling, or hiking. To find peace, to find purpose in life, to replace an addiction or bad habit with something healthier, to supplant emotional anguish with physical strength—these are all reasons to pursue endurance sports.

During endurance events, athletes deal with intense fatigue, dehydration, weather, physical obstacles such as hills, and if the race lasts longer than twenty-four hours, sleep deprivation. Pair that with negative thoughts and feelings of self-doubt, and it sounds like pure misery. But it comes down to mind over matter: If you can accept fatigue and push through the moments you feel like quitting, you can reach a goal that you never thought possible. And *that* can feel enjoyable.

The limbic system responds to immediate rewards, but the prefrontal cortex thrives on achieving long-term goals. Each time you complete a goal and reach the finish line, the prefrontal cortex gets a little bit stronger, and so does your determination and will. You push harder the next time, and the next unattainable goal comes closer into view, until it seems within reach.

Certain personality traits, such as having a type A personality or being goal-oriented and driven, can contribute to the development of eating disorders. But they can also be used in a positive way to fuel athletic performance. According to a 2018 study in *Psychology of Sport and Exercise* that examined the minds of ultramarathoners, the most motivating factor for ultrarunners is the opportunity to achieve a personal goal, not losing weight or achieving a lean physique.[30] Ultrarunners are intrinsically motivated by a desire to achieve something great and explore their mental and physical limits.

The short-term effects are fatigue and muscle soreness, but the long-lasting effects are feeling powerful and taking pride in one's mental and physical toughness. Not the hubristic pride that comes from social media likes or compliments about being skinny, but authentic pride in who you are and your ability to conquer challenges—the kind of pride that comes from enduring and emerging stronger in the end. For me, ultrarunning is a reminder that my body can achieve so much more than I ever gave it credit for and that I can make it to any finish line if I put my mind to it.

Running is my drug, my cross-addiction, a healthy substitute for an unhealthy habit. It keeps me sane when life is stressful. Running has taught me to love my body again, something I forgot how to do for years. I feel beautiful after a run, when I'm achy and drenched in sweat. While I know running is good for me—there are proven benefits for cardiovascular health, bone health, and prevention of diabetes and other metabolic diseases—that is not why I am hooked. A blood pressure of 110/70 and a high-density lipoprotein level of 99 are good for my heart, but my heart doesn't love running. My mind does. I choose to run again and again. Why do I keep coming back for more? How does my brain make an activity that some consider torturous feel pleasurable?

Most people are familiar with the term "runner's high," a mythical euphoric state associated with running. Even non-

15 | EXERCISE JUNKIE

runners, people who say they "only run if I'm being chased," have heard of it. But most runners never experience a high, regardless of how far or how often they run. Instead, they feel calm, less anxious, and more relaxed during and after a run. They experience a "flow state" in which they are fully absorbed in the act of running itself, reaching a state of mindfulness despite the physical challenge of constant movement. It is the same way an artist gets lost in a painting, a Buddhist monk meditates for hours despite the physical discomfort of sitting in one place, or a writer burns through twenty pages of prose without even sipping their coffee. Flow state is "being in the zone" or "going on autopilot."

Runners can enter a flow state because running activates endogenous opioids and endocannabinoids, substances that make the activity feel enjoyable and their minds feel focused. Endocannabinoids are molecules that act on the same system activated by tetrahydrocannabinol (THC), the active compound in cannabis. They can boost mood both during and after a run, sometimes to the point of euphoria, but more often they create a feeling of calm and lessened anxiety. Like endogenous opioids, also called endorphins, they have an analgesic effect, dulling the sensation of pain that comes with prolonged exercise. This is one reason runners can push past the wall—the 20-mile mark in a marathon when your body runs out of glycogen, your muscles feel like a pile of bricks, and no amount of Tylenol or Advil can save you—and keep moving for another six miles in pursuit of the finish line.

In general, exercise boosts brain health and the body's response to stress, not only through the release of endocannabinoids and endorphins, but also through serotonin, dopamine, norepinephrine, and oxytocin—the same neurotransmitters that become unbalanced in eating disorders and mood disorders. But unlike using a drug like oxycodone or marijuana to mitigate pain, or using an SSRI to treat depression, exercise is a natural way to enhance neurotransmitters in just the right increments, without unwanted side effects or cravings. Exercise is a way to restore homeostasis.

These chemical changes in the brain occur while moving, but there are long-lasting effects on brain health that extend beyond the period of physical activity. Have you ever noticed how you feel sharper and happier after a workout? That is not due merely to a sense of accomplishment at doing something physically challenging; animal models show that exercise increases blood flow to the brain and induces neurogenesis, the process of creating new neurons, in the hippocampus, which enhances processes related to memory and learning. Exercise can improve cognitive processes, such as focused thinking, attention span, emotional regulation, and perception.

In fact, the majority of people who exercise do it for mental health and emotional well-being as much as for physical fitness. Exercise is self-motivating, self-powered, and more affordable and accessible than psychotherapy. The American Psychological Association even considers movement a second-line therapy for the treatment of depression. According to a 2022 review in the *Journal of Affective Disorders*, exercise combined with standard treatments like therapy and medication led to significantly greater antidepressant effects in study patients.[31] Other studies have shown that one in nine cases of depression could potentially be prevented if all adults did 150 minutes of moderate-intensity physical activity per week, which is the minimal amount recommended by the US Centers for Disease Control and Prevention.[32] Exercise has yet to become medicalized, but when it does, I will gladly write a prescription for it.

Every time I run, my brain bathes in a slurry of mood-enhancing chemicals. While I have never felt a runner's high, the effects of a long-distance run on my mood and stress level are reproducible and indisputable. After the first few miles, running starts to feel easier, not harder. My breathing is unlabored, and my muscles are pliable and relaxed. Aches and pains are muted. Each step flows into the next with a steady rhythm. My body switches to cruise control and I feel like I can keep going forever. My mind drifts and sometimes goes silent, a break from the constant mental chatter of everyday life. Afterward, I feel peaceful and content. I seek that feeling of tranquility over and over.

My brain likes to spin on the hamster wheel. I have replaced one habit (bingeing and purging) with another (habitual exercise). Instead of feeling shameful and bloated after a binge, I feel mentally and physically healthy after a run. Running has become a part of who I am, integral to my happiness. But as someone who has struggled with mental health issues and engaged in self-destructive behaviors, I have to ask myself: Am I an exercise junkie? Do I truly love running as much as I think I do, or am I addicted to it?

We can become dependent on activities the same way we do with substances. Signs of dependence include building up a tolerance and needing increasing amounts of an activity to get the desired effect; withdrawing from recreational and social functions to get that activity; and physical and mental withdrawal symptoms that occur when we suddenly stop doing it.

When I can't run for a few days, I feel its absence. I get irritable, restless, bored. I can kickbox or use an elliptical at the gym, but there is no substitute for running. Any other activity is a watered-down version of the exercise my body craves, the nicotine gum for the chain-smoker. And sometimes a quick three-mile run is not enough; I need an hour of running to put me at ease. When I'm tired, I convince myself to run anyway, knowing it will make me feel better in the end. What would I do if an injury or illness took away my ability to run? Would I be able to cope with the loss? Or would I throw the crutches aside, skip the follow-up appointment, and hobble along on a broken bone or torn ligament, driven by the need to run? I am not sure. I would like to think my prefrontal cortex would know better, after all I have been through. But, as they say, doctors make the worst patients.

Chapter 16

A NEW HIGH

"Are you sure you're going to be safe? Do you know what you're doing up there?" my mom asked. I was thirty-seven years old, but she was still my mom, trying to protect me from the world. "I promise I'll be careful. That's why I'm climbing with a group. If I fall in a crevasse, someone will be there to pull me out!" I said, half joking. She was not amused. My mom was the risk-averse, cautious parent, the one who told me to be safe walking home from work in Philly and driving in snow in Denver. She cringed when I signed up for ultramarathons, afraid I would get injured. But I was adventurous, a trait I inherited from my dad, which only made it less endearing to her. She didn't understand why I wanted to mountaineer.

She asked me a series of questions: Where would I be sleeping? Did I pack enough clothes? Did I remember a toothbrush? Each question was a reminder as I packed my 65-liter backpack with mountaineering gear: ice axe, crampons, trekking poles, a zero-degree sleeping bag, carabiners, glacier goggles, climbing harness, headlamp, and La Sportiva climbing boots that cost more than Louboutin pumps. It was a 35-pound jigsaw puzzle with each item fitted perfectly into place.

The Mount Rainier trip was a three-day climb along the Disappointment Cleaver Route, the easiest and most commonly traveled route for new mountaineers. But it would still be a grueling climb across snow and ice, with hazards like crevasses, rockfall, and loose volcanic scree along the way. The climb touched the Cowlitz and Emmons Glaciers, two of the massive glaciers covering the slopes of the mountain. Regardless of the route, and there are many, Mount Rainier is considered the toughest climb in the Lower 48 states. It is a training ground for people who want to tackle bigger glaciated peaks outside the US; what it lacks in height, it makes up for in ferocity. Winter and early spring snowstorms can trap climbers on the mountain, leaving them with no chance of reaching the top, and avalanches and crevasses have taken many lives over the years. Only 50 percent of summit attempts are successful. So why was I going to climb it? I had to ask myself the same question.

It started with a documentary. Rich and I were relaxing at home and browsing Netflix when we came across *14 Peaks: Nothing Is Impossible*. We watched Nims Purja and his team of Nepalese climbers summit the fourteen tallest peaks in the world in record-breaking time. I was immediately enthralled. I had seen the grandeur of the Rocky Mountains, but the beastly snow-covered peaks in the documentary, including Mount Everest, were even more awe-inspiring. My pulse quickened and my palms started to sweat (thanks, amygdala) as I watched the climbers push through strong headwinds and snow squalls into the "death zone" above 8,000 meters. I leaned forward in my seat, inching closer to the TV screen. It was gripping; I had never had such a visceral reaction to a documentary before.

The next time we curled up together on the couch, Rich said, "Let's watch this one about K2." He clicked play on the remote, clearly interested too. "Would you ever try this?" I asked, pupils dilating as images of the snowy pyramid filled the screen. He answered with a casual yes. "I would," I said with conviction, as if I had already booked a flight to Pakistan for the next expedition. We watched as many mountaineering and rock-climbing documentaries as we could find, and I read just as many books about conquering huge peaks and granite walls under the worst conditions: unpredictable storms, frigid temperatures, frostbite, crevasse rescues, high-altitude cerebral edema, surviving in the death zone when bottled oxygen ran out. *No Shortcuts to the Top* by Ed Viesturs, *Into Thin Air* by Jon Krakauer, *Touching the Void* by Joe Simpson, *The Girl Who Climbed Everest* by Bonita Norris— the list went on. At night I dreamed of the mountains and awoke with a feverish longing to climb them, the same way I had dreamt about food when I was starving.

Could I become a mountaineer? Mountaineering combined hiking and adventure, two things I loved. Just like ultrarunning, it welcomed anyone willing to try it, indifferent to age or gender. Every mountaineering podcast I listened to claimed that "strong legs and big lungs" were the key to success. I had both. If I could use them to run long distances without ever feeling breathless, maybe I could use them on a mountain. Mountaineering would test my endurance in a different way, without the overuse injuries and recurrent aches and pains that came with constantly pounding pavement as a runner. Thankfully I had never suffered a real injury, but I knew that running marathons, and ultras, could exact a toll on my body.

But becoming a mountaineer was an unconventional goal. It

wasn't part of the linear path I was used to following: student to doctor, girlfriend to wife, 5K to marathon. It was a leap in a completely new direction, from suburban New Jersey to the summit of a glaciated mountain. I felt inexplicably drawn to the mountains. What would I find there? Would reaching a summit fulfill my need to achieve in the same way that getting straight A's or running an ultramarathon did? While I was no longer anorexic, I was still goal oriented. Or maybe I was just seeking novelty and danger. As a recovered binge eater, I could appreciate the rush of pleasure and excitement that came with doing something risky. Skydiving, rappelling, white water rafting, ice climbing—I had tried them all. My brain loved a good dopamine fix. Was I just an exercise junkie looking for another cross-addiction? Or was I trying to find myself in nature, the same way I had when I hiked in Colorado as an adult or the Appalachian Trail as a kid? I had to find out.

But I'm not *stupid*. I had learned my lesson about preparation. Before I dove into mountaineering headfirst, I dipped my toes in shallow water. I signed up for my first official guided climb on Mount Baker. A heavily glaciated stratovolcano, Mount Baker ranks third among the highest peaks in Washington State at a height of 10,781 feet, providing a picturesque background for the town of Bellingham. After Mount Rainier, it has the heaviest glacial coverage of the Cascade Range volcanoes, and it is the second-most thermally active crater after Mount St. Helens. It is also the perfect training ground for an aspiring mountaineer. The requirements to climb were a good fitness level and a laundry list of gear. Fitness I had; the rest I could buy. I flew out to Seattle in mid-September and met the International

Mountain Guides (IMG) group, an all-female team consisting of two guides and one other climber, on the first morning of our expedition.

I was the only one wearing mascara, hair neatly pulled back, skin scented with vanilla perfume—the way I usually presented myself when not trail running with dirt caked on my shins. The guides were gritty and—based on the climbing gear, ropes, and thin mattresses splayed out in the back seats—seemed to live out of their hatchback cars. Angie, one of the guides, was energetic and lanky, with a blonde ponytail that matched mine. She was following in the footsteps of her dad, who was also a mountaineer, and she had recently guided her first attempt on Denali. Lindsey, native to Philadelphia, had the witty, sharp personality of an East Coaster, and sturdy, muscular legs from constant mountain guiding and trail running. Brie was the only other climber who had signed up, and she had just completed a climb of Mount St. Helens. She was an experienced backpacker and camper and looked like the poster child for REI.

I suddenly felt out of place and inexperienced, with the anxiety of an insecure teenager about to be rejected by the popular girls again. Being a jock was the only thing that had saved me from ridicule in high school, but on this team of athletic women, I was the girly girl. I didn't even know how to use a cookstove or put on crampons.

When we set out on the first day in hiking boots, my upper body sagged under the weight of the 30-pound pack on my shoulders. Every step jostled the pack, straining my shoulders and neck. I was all legs, the ultramarathon runner who couldn't do push-ups. I wasn't sure if I could keep up with the others. But no one cared about the speed of the ascent; they cared about enjoying the journey. They were friendly and chatty, talking about previous climbs, adventures, trail running, and hiking. We had plenty of things in common. As we hiked farther and farther from civilization, the anxieties of everyday life seemed to melt away. The Mount Baker wilderness was an untouched world without commotion, traffic, or cell service; instead, it had sweeping views of the valley below and the invigorating smell of conifer trees.

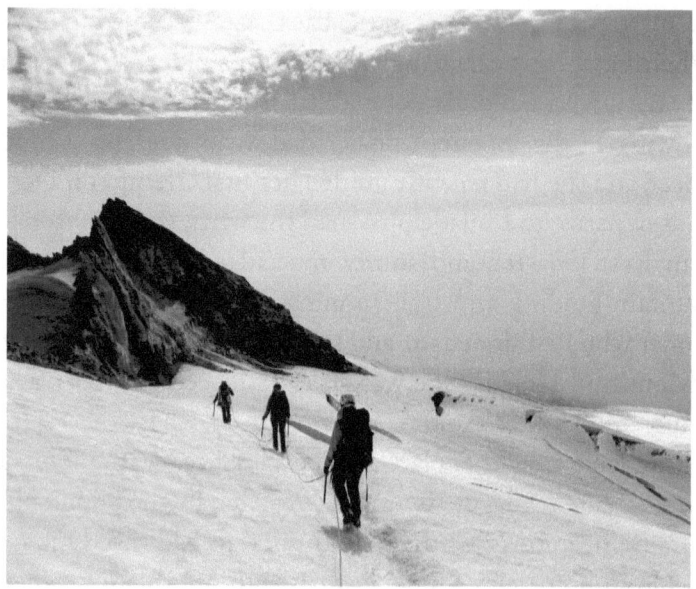

Mount Baker

Camp was set up on a small outcropping of rocks at the base of the glacier. Next to our tents was the glacial runoff, a small stream of ice-cold water for drinking and cooking. The constant flow of water past our tents, nature's white noise machine, helped us drift off to sleep at night. Instead of staring at our phones in the evening, we watched everything around us. We were a part of the landscape: the sun setting over the North Cascades, the glistening lake below camp, ducks and furry marmots scurrying across the rocks, and four women, bundled up in parkas, sipping tea and hot cocoa made from boiled snowmelt. It was a simple and beautiful way of existing.

Why hadn't I camped before? I had missed out on so much in my twenties, unaware of the healing effects of nature while I served time in the city, imprisoned by residency and mental health struggles, surrounded by millions of strangers and high-rise buildings. In my thirties, there were many times I could have camped after a long solo hike in the Rockies, many places I could have watched the stars or fallen asleep to the sound of running water from inside my sleeping bag—I just didn't know to. It was time to buy a tent.

On summit day, we awoke at 4:30 a.m. and crept out of our tents. The night had transformed the surrounding rocks and sky into a purple-hued moonscape. I put on my mountaineering boots and carefully laced up my crampons, following the instructions of the guides, until they were tight around the heels and toes of my boots. We started up toward the frosty tongue of the Easton Glacier, each step marked by the grating crunch of crampons on boulders. Lacing crampons, tying knots, using an ice axe to self-arrest during a fall—these were basic but invaluable skills, and I practiced them on the snowy slopes of Mount Baker.

As we marched along, the rocky moonscape turned into a maze of chunky blue ice at the bottom of the glacier and then finally into a smooth incline of wind-scalloped snow. Tiny crevasses were everywhere, as if the surface of the glacier had been slashed with a knife. We stepped across them without looking down, terrified by the deep blue-black hue of the void below. Clouds drifted across the Cascades, dousing us with raindrops as we hurriedly pulled on hard shell jackets and pants. But as soon as we finished piling on clothes, the rain stopped. Daylight broke, the morning haze cleared, and layers upon layers of mountains became visible in the distance. They looked like an acrylic painting, with dark, angular bursts of blue and gray in the foreground and hazy, snowy brushstrokes in the background. Beyond that, the horizon was a cloudless cobalt hue.

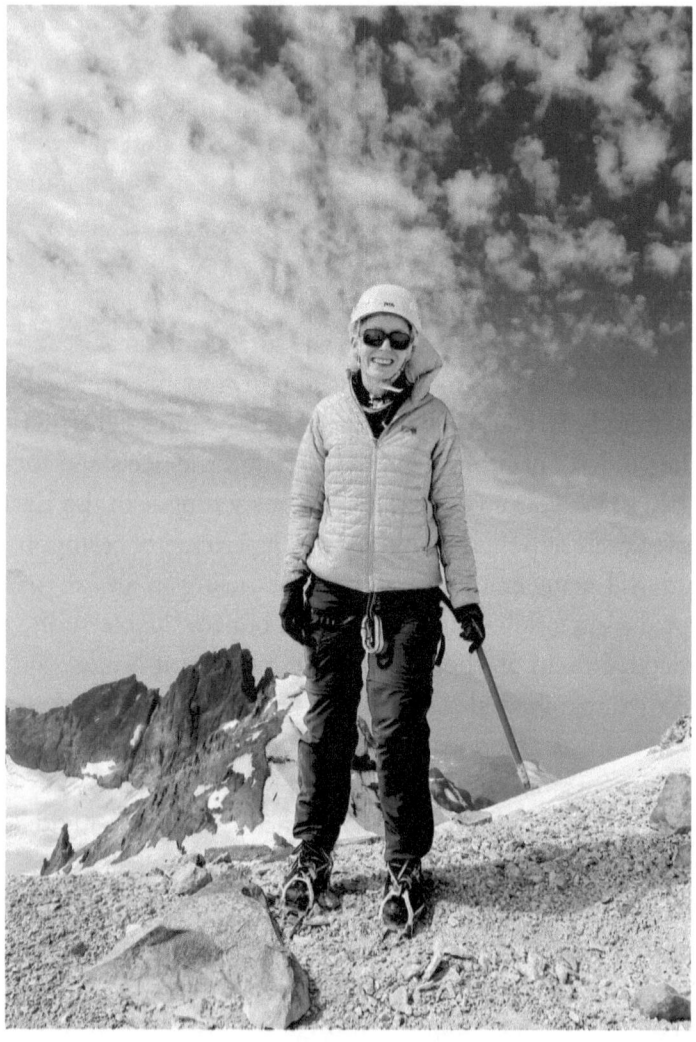

Summit of Mount Baker

"How do you feel?" Lindsey asked seven hours later as we crested the top of the volcano. "Isn't it beautiful up here?" I breathed in the pungent smell of sulfur emanating from the caldera as I took in the views. "I'm exhausted!" I replied, falling in a heap onto the snow and rock. My legs felt as heavy as the boulders. "But I can see why you love it. I'd stay here forever if I could." The view from the crater was beautiful, and the journey to get there had been challenging but somehow more rewarding than the summit itself. Mountaineering was the sister of endurance running; it required sustained focus and stamina. It was Type II fun, and I wanted to do it again. "You should sign up for our Mount Rainier climb next time," she said. "It's a lot tougher than this, but you'll love it." It didn't take much convincing; I signed up for the expedition as soon as I got home.

We started our descent back to camp, sloshing and sliding on snow softened by the afternoon sun. My heart felt light as my feet plowed through the slush. I thought back to the unanswered question: Why climb the mountain? I still wasn't sure. I loved the climb without caring about the summit. I never felt like my life was in danger. Maybe I needed the mountains to give me peace, as they had when I hiked in Rocky Mountain National Park. Maybe I needed them to keep me honest, to remind me to never let my health and vitality slip away again. Maybe Mount Rainier would have the answer I was looking for. That night I burrowed into my sleeping bag, tired and content, beneath a ceiling of stars. I drifted off, listening to the wind and the wisdom of the mountain, and slept the deepest sleep of my life.

Chapter 17

ABOVE THE CLOUDS

Don't look down, I told myself. My headlamp illuminated a precipitous, unforgiving drop mere feet away. Even in the dark, I knew there were jagged rocks and a crevasse directly below, a dangerous place to fall. It was as hard to look up as down, my view of the stars obscured by a helmet and headlamp that kept slipping down across my forehead. Instead, I focused on the boots of the guide in front of me and tried to copy his steps, wedging the toe of my crampon into cracks between the rocks. His movements were dance-like and precise; mine were teetering and off-balance, made clumsier by the weight of the pack pulling me backward. Crampons were meant for snow, and trying to gain traction on loose rocks and ash made each step feel more awkward than the last. It was strange to feel unsteady on my feet, the same sturdy feet that had carried me through multiple marathons.

We were slowly making our way up the Disappointment Cleaver, a lengthy, steep rock ridge separating the Ingraham and Emmons Glaciers on Mount Rainier. We traversed the spine of it for two hours before regaining footing on the upper part of the

Emmons Glacier. For me, it was the crux of the climb; it was not technical, just punishing and relentless. Every step forward resulted in a slide back. It was a massive jungle gym of boulders and scree. Some boulders were too large to step over, so I climbed them, crampons and ice pick creaking as they dug into solid rock. The friction created sparks that popped off the spikes of my crampons, like tiny fireworks on a starry Fourth of July night.

Progress up the Disappointment Cleaver, nicknamed "the DC," was arduous, the way marked by small reflective wands that had been twisted into the rock to form a path. Every wand we passed put us a few steps closer to the top, a never-ending game of connect-the-dots. We were short-roping, tied together in groups of three with only a few feet of taut rope between us. Step too far, and you rammed into the person in front of you; step short, and you got dragged along, the weakest link in the chain. Short-roping was a safety measure, but a climber's fall could create a domino effect, ripping the other climbers off the ridge. The guides were trusting us as much as we were trusting them.

My heart rate quickened, and my muscles tensed. I had always had a fear of falling off an edge—driving over mountain passes, standing on the rim of the Grand Canyon, and even looking off the side of a ski lift scared me—and this was testing my limits. Again, I wondered if climbing was satisfying some impulsive need to take a risk, to do something daring. Was I really in danger, or was it just fear, my brain's response to something that *seemed* scary? Fear was the limbic system's cry for attention, a sign that it was in fight-or-flight mode. On the DC, it was hard to see the line separating danger and fear, especially shrouded in darkness. I chose to keep moving forward. Tonight was the summit bid, and I was not about to turn back.

17 | ABOVE THE CLOUDS

Three days earlier, I had arrived in Ashford, Washington, the launchpad for Mount Rainier climbing expeditions, just miles away from the Paradise entrance to Mount Rainier National Park. It was the first day of August, and the weather was perfect— 80°F with sunny, clear blue skies. Higher up the mountain, the temperature would plummet and the winds would pick up. And there was always a chance of rain and thunderstorms. The mountain was mercurial, and it would decide whether we summited or not.

Avalanches were less of a concern in late summer, but crevasses and collapsing snow bridges still posed a risk. The tallest peak in the Cascade Range, Mount Rainier stands at 14,410 feet and is covered by an extensive system of approximately two dozen glaciers (the number has decreased in recent years due to climate change) and over thirty-five square miles of snowfields. The most topographically prominent mountain in the contiguous United States, it looms over Seattle from a distance, inspiring awe as well as a sense of foreboding. Because of its proximity to nearby towns and homes, it is considered one of the most dangerous volcanoes in the world.

My fascination with the mountain grew each time I saw it. My first view was through the corner of an airplane window, when the pilot pointed out its snowy cap above the clouds— the closest most people would come to seeing Rainier's summit. Then I saw it from Seattle, a massive white dome glowing in the setting sun, as I dined at a waterfront seafood restaurant where I had intentionally chosen the seat with a mountain view. After climbing Mount Baker, I visited Mount Rainier National Park to get a closer look at the volcano. The mountain is only visible about eighty days out of the year, but I had seen it every time I visited the Pacific Northwest. It flaunted its beauty invitingly. *I'll be back to climb you,* I promised.

The only place I could not see Mount Rainier was in Ashford, a mere five miles from the entrance to the park. Douglas firs and cedar trees cocooned the small town, eclipsing any views of the mountain. The climbing team, made up of seven men and four guides from IMG, piled into a small van to be transported to the trailhead. I sized up the other climbers; I would be sharing sleeping space with a group of guys I didn't know. Mountaineering was still a boys' club, and I was the only woman who had signed up. It felt like I was back on the boys' traveling soccer team, having to prove my worth as an athlete. Or worse, having to prove myself as a young female resident, when I was constantly demoted to nurse or student. I hated being underestimated, but it made me want to work harder.

"What training did you do for this?" Greg asked, offering me a handful of jelly beans as the van climbed along the road to Paradise. Greg was a "highpointer" tackling one of the hardest high points in the US; he had daughters close to my age, and I came to see him as a father figure. "I climbed Mount Baker last year, and I've run a few ultramarathons," I replied. "I'll never be able to keep up with you!" another climber chimed in, showing deference. Maybe they would accept me into the pack.

The men were of varying ages and climbing backgrounds; one had trekked to Everest base camp, another had climbed Mount St. Helens, and a father-son team had attempted to climb Mount Rainier two years earlier, only to get trapped at camp for five days in a late spring snowstorm. Now we shared a common goal—to make it to the top—and we would need each other to get there. The van buzzed with conversation, as if we were a group of kids sharing the bus on the first day of school.

The trailhead was bustling with park rangers and tourists ambling along the paved parts of the Skyline Trail. Mount Rainier stood in the distance, a snow-capped king reigning over

17 | ABOVE THE CLOUDS

a realm of beauty; in the foreground were clusters of wildflowers—scarlet paintbrush, alpine aster, lupine, and mountain heather. We started the six-hour hike to Camp Muir and I started sweating immediately, baking beneath the brilliant sunlight. The sun intensified the higher we climbed, from pavement to dirt to subalpine meadows and eventually to the Muir Snowfield, a two-mile stretch of snow that reflected the light back up at our glacier goggles.

Now I know why they told me to put sunscreen on my lips and up my nose. There was no hiding from the sun on the Muir Snowfield; it was above the snowline, the altitude at which snow remains unmelted through the summer and the fir trees and mountain hemlock that grow at lower elevations disappear. The heat and constant stomping of other hikers turned the snow into soft serve ice cream by midday and made each step feel harder under the weight of heavy packs. But once we reached Camp Muir, the hikers turned back, and the mountain belonged to the mountaineers. Camp Muir, once named Cloud Camp, sits at an elevation of about 10,200 feet and consists of a few century-old buildings, including a guide hut and a shelter for climbers.

"Is anyone else going to watch the sunset?" I zipped up my parka and put gloves on. The night air had already chilled to 50°F. "If you're going, I'll go," said Kyle, grabbing his camera, and three others followed. Everyone else was already asleep in the climbers' hut, sleeping bags and mats rolled out on thin wooden platforms used as beds. I knew I needed rest for the next day, but I couldn't miss the incredible sunset.

The horizon turned into sherbet, with hazy shades of peach, crimson, and orange melting into each other. We could see the Tatoosh Range to the south and, beyond that, Mount Adams, Mount Hood, and Mount St. Helens glowing in the waning light. The volcanoes looked deceptively small in the vast, rugged landscape. As the sun sank and we fell into darkness, I snapped a few photos with my phone, then tucked it back in my pocket. We stood in silence, appreciating the view. *I wish my husband could see this*, I thought; he was three time zones away, sleeping soundly, and I vowed to bring him back on a future hiking trip. When the last drop of color faded from the sky, we retreated to our sleeping bags and settled in for the night.

The smell of chocolate chip pancakes and French-press coffee—the perfect cure for an altitude headache—greeted us in the cook tent the next morning. The guides made sure we were well fed at every meal and rest stop. "The best part of mountaineering is eating whatever you want, whenever you want," said Max, the lead guide. He had just returned from the summit of Mount Everest. I added "unlimited food" to the list of reasons to become a mountaineer. There was no room for dieting when you were pushing your body to extremes. We dug into breakfast as a team, shoulder to shoulder, despite our clothes smelling of yesterday's dried sweat, and then roped up to continue the ascent.

We traversed the Cowlitz Glacier on the way to high camp. It was littered with TV-sized boulders that had fallen from higher up, like the aftermath of a meteor strike. I suddenly saw rocks and dust careening toward us; we had to move fast to avoid being struck by anything bigger. We scrambled up Cathedral Gap, a stair-climber of loose ash and dirt. Each named segment of the climb seemed to offer a different challenge. Every forceful step made my head pound like a drum. My heart flip-flopped, and I wasn't sure if it was the altitude, the effort, or the strong coffee causing the palpitations.

High camp was on the Ingraham Flats at an elevation of over 11,000 feet, a cluster of five yellow tents and a basic cook tent perched on a snowfield. Precariously situated below camp was a crevasse large enough to swallow a house. The crevasses on Mount Rainier are deep, sometimes up to hundreds of feet, forming jagged, unstable tears in the upper layers of the glacier. We were reminded to stay within ten feet of camp at all times to avoid falling into any hidden crevasses. The jaws of the beast could open up anywhere.

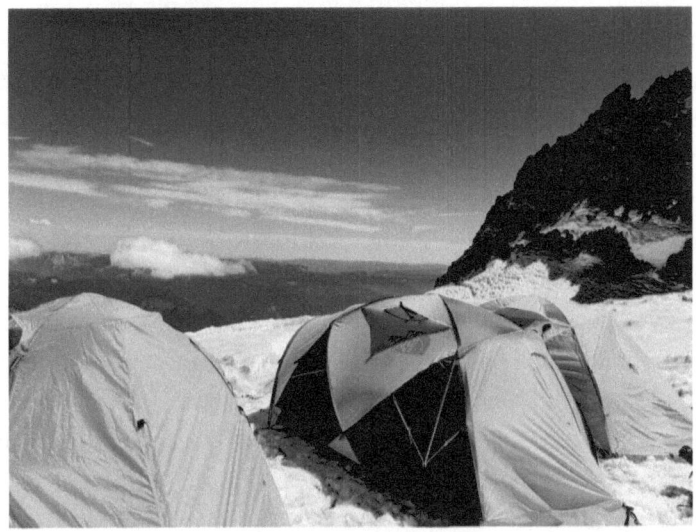

Mount Rainier high camp

Socks and shirts dried on the roofs of neon yellow tents under the afternoon sun as we sat down for an early dinner. With the summit push starting at 10:30 that night, we had only a few hours to rest before we would be up and climbing again. Max briefed us on the night ahead. "The summit is only halfway. The goal is not to come back down the mountain wasted, to be carried all the way back to the trailhead. The goal is to finish strong." The guides would make the ultimate decision about who would summit, and there was no room for argument. We all nodded. Quickly, his serious demeanor was replaced with a wide grin.

"Right on!" he said. "Now go get some sleep." Lying in my sleeping bag with the tent door open, I saw fluffy clouds below camp, layered over the triangular Little Tahoma Peak. It was my first cloud inversion, more beautiful than I had imagined.

A chorus of cell phone alarms sounded at exactly 10:30 p.m., a savage wake-up call. Day and night had been turned upside down, and we were waking up when most people were going to bed. Thankfully, years of overnight calls had prepared me well. I could wake up from a deep sleep and shake off grogginess with the snap of a finger. I sprang up from my sleeping bag and packed my backpack as if the tent were on fire. Outside in the frosty air, I used my headlamp and the celestial glow of the moon to quickly put on my harness and crampons.

The night sky was full of stars, the only spectators for our midnight climb. They watched as we started the summit bid, the overnight journey that would test our stamina and endurance and, we hoped, make us Mount Rainier summiteers. We were down to six climbers; two men willingly stayed at high camp, happy they had made it "far enough." But I could not imagine giving up now, when I was only six or seven hours from the summit. That was the duration of a 50K race, and I knew I could push through it.

"We're going to move as quickly as we can through this section. Even if you lose a crampon, DO NOT stop moving." There was a sense of urgency from the guides as we marched across the snow toward the Disappointment Cleaver. A serac loomed overhead, capable of dropping a piano-sized ice block on us at any moment.

We reached the first ladder crossing, a one-lane bridge that spanned a crevasse. We had to step carefully but efficiently across the rungs, with the only support being a rope we clipped into and used as a handrail. Luckily the crevasse's width was much

17 | ABOVE THE CLOUDS

less daunting than its depth. Looking down, there was a spectrum of color, ranging from brilliant blue untouched ice at the top to a thick, inky black where it became impossible to see the bottom. *What if my crampon gets stuck on a rung? What if I slip?* Walking across a horizontal ladder over a gaping hole terrified me. I gripped the anchored hand rope tightly, choked down my fear, and stepped onto the ladder, focused on keeping my balance. Each step was answered by a groaning sound as the metal rungs flexed beneath my weight. Only when I reached the other side did I remember to breathe. Then I hurriedly kept moving as instructed. There was no time for reflection.

At the top of the Disappointment Cleaver, I drank half a liter from my Nalgene bottle in one gulp. "Do you know why it's named the Disappointment Cleaver?" our guide Lindsey asked. "Because it sucks?!" Jason replied, short-roped behind me. I had to laugh and admit that it really did suck. I was exhausted, and we were nowhere near the top. The real answer was that one of the earliest climbing groups to ascend Rainier had gone up in a storm and, because of poor visibility, thought the top of the DC was the summit. In actuality, it fell about 2,000 feet short of the crater; the summit was still hours away.

Above the DC, the trail wound steadily like a sidewinder along the slope of the glacier, with sweeping views below and the glow of climbers' headlamps above. With every step and turn of a head, the light of the headlamps bounced and flickered like fireflies on a warm summer night. Far in the distance, we could see the city lights of Yakima. I studied the snow off to the side of the trail, noticing how the wind had swept it into patterns. At first it looked like a gentle tide frozen in place, with small bumpy waves scattered across the surface; then it was whipped into sugary peaks that resembled the top of a meringue pie; farther on, it became sharp and pointed like icy stalagmites. For an East Coaster who was used to a level pancake of snow coating the ground, the transformation was magical.

The next break did not come for another two hours, and my mouth was parched. I longed to reach down with my glove and grab a fresh fistful of snow to melt in my mouth, but I could not risk dropping my ice axe. One careless move could get me kicked off the climb. We were down to five; another climber could not maintain the pace. He looked dejected heading back to high camp. The Disappointment Cleaver, his turnaround point, seemed aptly named in that moment.

We finally stopped at "High Break," a resting point along the ridge at 13,500 feet of elevation. I leaned into the mountain, settled against my pack, and pulled out a snack. Cold air nipped at my fingertips. "Am I doing okay? Is my pace good enough?" I asked Matt, the guide at the head of my rope team. *Please don't tell me it's over. Let me make the summit.* As the only woman on the climb, would I be the next to be cut? "You're doing great," he said. "Don't worry—you are definitely making the summit!" Those words of reassurance were all I needed to hear to keep going.

Just 900 feet of elevation left to go until we reached the crater. My mind convinced me that the terrain was getting steeper, but maybe that was the altitude talking. I felt slightly foggy and hazy, and each step seemed more effortful. I listened to the tinny squeak of my ice axe spike digging into the crusty snow, like an overused shopping cart turning its wheels; even my crampons and ice axe were tired. I kept a slow but steady pace, using the mountaineer's rest step—a method in which you lock your back knee, putting all your weight on it and allowing your front leg to completely relax for a second—to give my calves momentary respite from the constant burn of lactic acid that was searing my muscles. Up ahead, Max called out, "Only ten minutes to go!" and we pressed on.

Ten minutes to go. *Powerful. Perseverance.* The mantra that kept me going in a marathon was just as motivating on a mountain. I had to dig deep and tap into the last stores of energy, will, and determination I could find. When my muscles wanted to stop, my brain told them to keep moving forward. It was a constant conversation, and then an argument, a battle between body and mind. But I knew which one would win. The ability to summit the mountain came down to drive and mental fortitude. Mountaineering, like ultrarunning, was a feat of endurance, fueled by a powerful connection with nature and a desire to test the limits of how far I could go.

My eyes were trained on the rope team ahead of me until they disappeared over the rocky lip of the crater. We were finally there. I took the last few steps up to the summit and into the crater as brilliant streaks of red, orange, and pink streamed across the skyline to herald the sunrise. "Holy shit! I'm on the summit of Mount Rainier!" I shouted above the wind, grinning from ear to ear. Huddled together on the crater, we exchanged gloved fist bumps and pats on the back in celebration. It was only 5:10 a.m.

Despite the wind chill of 10°F, the crater felt warm and eerily calm. I sank into the snow and relaxed, knowing the hardest part of the climb was over. It was the toughest physical challenge I had faced so far, and although I was tired, I felt like I had more to give. My legs could carry me to even higher peaks and across greater distances, if I willed them to. My body was capable, fit, and strong. Why had I spent so many years trying to be thin? Being fit was so much more rewarding. I silently thanked the mountain. Nature could never be conquered, but that day the mountain had let us reach its summit, and I felt like I belonged there.

The summit was only a brief moment in the journey; we still had to descend. My heart and lungs were grateful to no longer be climbing uphill, but my quads and feet were punished on the way down. Within minutes my legs felt like Jell-O, quivering and bending under the weight of my pack. Max's comment about finishing the climb strong stayed with me. I didn't want to be the person who was carried back to the base of the mountain; I wanted the tourists at the Paradise parking lot to look at me with awe, knowing I had made the summit—and also keep their distance since I smelled like a wild woodland animal. I craved a shower, but I knew that as soon as I was back in Seattle in a crisp, clean hotel room, I would miss the dirt and grime and adventure. My skin was lightly coated with dust where sweat had mixed with volcanic ash, the mountaineer becoming one with the mountain; I was reluctant to wash away the earthen souvenir it had given me.

The sun rose fully and lit up the snowy path, exposing the parts of the climb I had feared most. I saw the steep drop-offs along the flank of the volcano and the Disappointment Cleaver and was grateful I had ascended them in the dark with only a vague awareness of them. When we reached the Ingraham Flats, we were congratulated by the climbers and guides who had stayed back. It felt like we were home again, reunited with our teammates.

We continued down to the Muir Snowfield, where the afternoon sun again turned the snow to slush; instead of taking slippery steps, we skied and skated with our boots on, then sat down and glissaded across the snow. It was an ocean of glistening white that seemed to stretch on forever. After fifteen hours on my feet, I was happy to let the snow carry me downhill.

The trailhead finally came into view, and only at the end of the journey did I let my body submit to exhaustion. We threw down our packs and collapsed into the van heading back to IMG headquarters. The only sound on the ride back was the hum of the air-conditioning and the snores of the men who had swiftly fallen asleep. I laid my head against the window, looked back at Mount Rainier one last time, and closed my eyes. It was the end of one adventure, but it would lead to bigger ones. I had turned my mountaineering fever dreams into a reality, and I wasn't going to stop now.

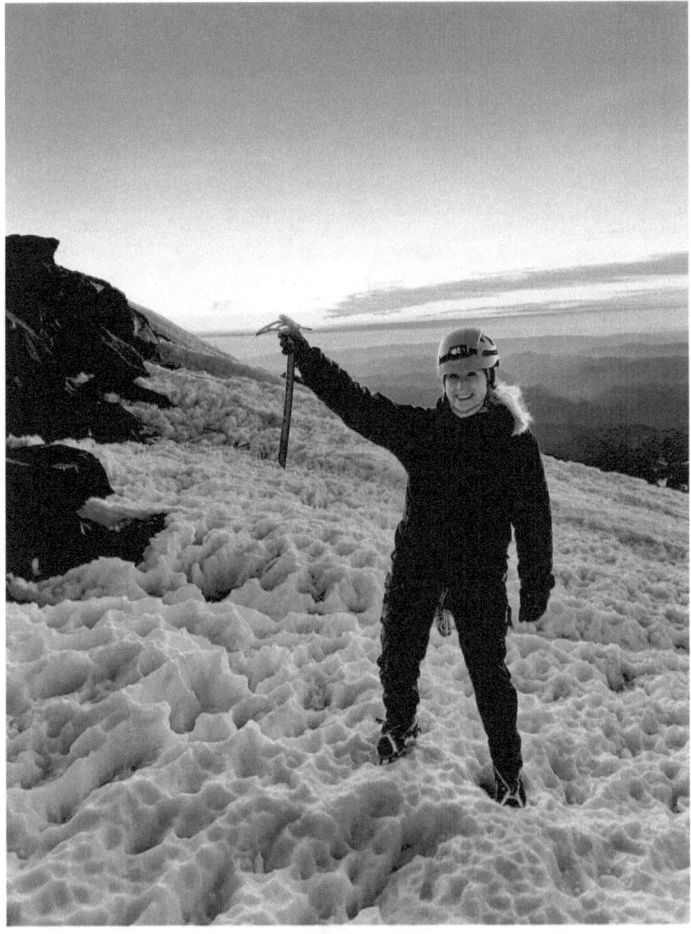

Summit of Mount Rainier

Chapter 18

INTO THE FOREST I GO

"And into the forest I go, to lose my mind and find my soul." One of my favorite John Muir quotes is probably a misquote. In fact, it's possible he never said or wrote any such thing. My real quibble with it, though, is that while we can lose our minds in nature (and I say that in a positive way), we can find them as well.

When I moved to Philadelphia as a resident, the city was exciting. Neon signs, colorful storefronts, the rich smell of Italian food wafting from restaurant doors. It teemed with life, people and cars marching like armies of ants along congested one-way streets. For someone in their twenties, the city held the promise of something new and exciting every day. But the longer I lived there, weighed down by depression and bulimia, the less charming the city became. Instead of fun, it was hectic and chaotic; the noises went from loud to deafening, and the smells went from aromatic to sour. My anxiety heightened with the frenetic pace of the city. Urban life had a hugely negative impact on my mental well-being, but I did not realize it until I had recovered many years later.

Living in Denver did not have the same effect, because I escaped the city every chance I got. I drove away to explore state parks, sparsely populated gold mining towns, highway exits that followed dirt roads and ended in trailheads. Outside of Denver, Colorado's only major city, the state was green space, open fields, dense forests, rushing streams, cerulean skies, and beautiful layers of hills and mountains. It was peaceful. Even the wildlife—bull elk roaming in Rocky Mountain National Park and pikas scurrying across hiking trails—looked content. I traded in urban life for nature, and my mental health rebounded swiftly. I credited my recovery to running and eventually mountaineering, sports I came to love because of my time in Colorado. But I sometimes wonder: If I had stayed in Colorado and simply *existed*, without becoming an endurance athlete, would nature have healed me anyway?

More than half the world's population lives in urban areas; this proportion is expected to rise to more than two-thirds by 2050. In the United States, that threshold has already been passed. While urban life typically offers better opportunities for jobs and housing and better access to healthcare, it also comes with negative effects on mental and physical health. A frequently cited study, published in *Acta Psychiatrica Scandinavica*, reported that people who live in cities are 21 percent more likely to have anxiety and 39 percent more likely to have depression than those in smaller towns and rural areas.[33] Living in a city can provoke a biologic stress response in the body, which leads not only to an increased risk of cardiovascular disease, stroke, and cancer, but also psychological symptoms such as anxiety, irritability, and depressed mood. It can make even a laid-back person feel high-strung. Surrounded by thousands or hundreds of thousands or even millions of other people, we feel uneasy, uncomfortable, and surprisingly alone.[34]

In urban settings, more time is spent indoors—sedentary, on screens, disengaged from nature, and disconnected from the world beyond the grid of city blocks in which we live. Physical activity has shifted indoors to gyms and home gym equipment, and prior to the COVID pandemic, over 50 percent of Americans didn't go outside for any recreation at all.[35] For those who want to play sports and exercise outdoors, rapid urbanization and less green space make it all the more difficult. I never ventured out to find a hiking or running trail outside Philadelphia, because it was too much work to leave the city. As a young woman, running alone through city parks risked my safety. And when I ran on crowded sidewalks, I was constantly annoyed by bumping elbows with strangers and stopping for traffic lights. It was much easier to stay confined to the gym, running in place on the same loop of treadmill belt. But it went against my love of nature, something engrained in me from the first time my soccer cleats touched fresh grass.

Nature and Mental Health

Urbanicity goes against the biophilia hypothesis, the concept that humans have an innate tendency to seek connection with nature and the living world. We are born to love nature because we evolved in it, and we find comfort in the sights, sounds, smells, and even the colors of the natural world. Being in nature can evoke feelings of peace, freedom, and even spirituality. Every person can benefit on an individual level, sometimes in entirely different ways, from being exposed to nature. This concept is not new. Over one hundred years ago, naturalist and explorer John Muir wrote (a verified quote!):

> Thousands of tired, nerve-shaken, over-civilized people are beginning to find out that going to the mountains is going

home; that wildness is a necessity; and that mountain parks and reservations are useful not only as fountains of timber and irrigating rivers, but as fountains of life.

Today, there is a growing body of evidence that supports Muir's observation and proves how much nature can positively impact health. You need not exercise to reap the benefits. Simply *being* in nature can induce physiologic changes that protect against the same diseases that cause chronic illness and mortality in tired, nerve-shaken, over-civilized city dwellers. A 2018 study published in *Health & Place* entailed a review of over forty experimental studies and showed that exposure to nature decreases stress levels based on measurements of heart rate, blood pressure, and cortisol, the body's primary stress hormone.[36] Participants in the studies reported feeling less stressed, a perceived effect on mood that mirrored the measurable changes in the body. Being in nature has been associated with happiness, positive affect, decreased anxiety, decreased depression, and an improved ability to manage stress and life tasks. The effects on mental health are often unmeasurable but even more profound than the effects on physical health.

Forty years ago, while Americans were witnessing the beginning of an obesity epidemic, the Japanese were focusing on a nature-based practice that demonstrated all these effects and more: *shinrin-yoku*, or forest bathing. The idea of forest bathing is to sit or slowly walk through the woods and completely immerse yourself in nature. If you are working too hard, like trail running or hiking, you are not forest bathing. Japanese studies of forest bathing showed that in both healthy people and those chronically ill with cardiac and renal disease, forest bathing not only lowered blood pressure and heart rate, but also improved blood sugar levels, improved sleep quality, decreased fatigue, lessened symptoms of anxiety and depression, and boosted immune system function. Improved immunity was due to phytoncides, natural oils emitted by trees that give them a fragrant smell and provide defense against insects and microbes; for humans, these substances increase levels of anti-inflammatory cytokines, natural killer cells, and proteins that can protect against cancer. Alpha-pinene, produced by conifer trees, is one well-known example of these compounds. It's no wonder we're drawn to the scent of pine and cedar.

Nature has cognitive benefits too. In everyday life, focused attention can be mentally taxing. Think of commuting to work in traffic, listening to meetings, and responding to emails while trying to drown out irrelevant background noise, and the digital fatigue that comes from spending too much time on devices toggling back and forth between apps, emails, and text messages. Sustaining attention and switching between different mental tasks is exhausting. When you immerse yourself in a restorative natural environment, you take a "mental break," and this can lower your perceived level of stress. In forest bathing, the goal is to reach a state of soft fascination, where the mind involuntarily absorbs the sights and sounds of nature and takes a break from focused attention on smartphone screens and noise. Evidence that we are indeed taking a mental break comes from functional magnetic resonance imaging (fMRI) studies and electroencephalography (EEG), two modalities that are used to study what is happening in the brain. When people look at natural rather than urban imagery, there is an increase in alpha brain waves, a type of brain wave that indicates an awake but relaxed state.[37]

In adults, forest bathing can improve working memory, cognitive flexibility, decision making, and impulse control, the same things that feel muddled when we are overly stressed. When we return to our daily tasks after spending time in nature, we are better equipped to handle them. Viewing a natural landscape—

even a brief glimpse of the color green—rather than staring at a smartphone screen, can enhance creative performance.[38] When we see something grander than a field of grass or a park—say, a majestic snow-covered mountain—we experience awe, a complex emotion that evokes feelings of wonder and amazement and makes our jaws drop as we simply say "wow." Individuals who experience awe in a positive way, as related to aesthetic natural scenery, score higher on creative thinking tests and also report higher rates of happiness and lower anxiety.

And in children, access to nature can improve school performance, foster imagination, and even improve attention in children with attention-deficit/hyperactivity disorder (ADHD). American kids do not go outside as much as they used to, and increased rates of depression, obesity, and vitamin D deficiency have been linked to this aptly nicknamed "nature deficit disorder." Even small doses of nature can make a difference. One study had a group of students stop in the middle of a monotonous, attention-draining task on a computer screen to look out the window. Students who looked at a flowering green roof for forty seconds made significantly fewer typing mistakes when they went back to the task, as compared to students who looked at a concrete roof.[39]

All these findings suggest that nature can nourish the prefrontal cortex, the brain's CEO. And nature exposure can come in many forms—it need not involve all the senses at once. Exposure to even one element of nature—the scent of pine or eucalyptus, an audio recording of waves crashing on the shore, a photograph of a beautiful landscape—can have beneficial effects on mental health. Multiple experimental studies have looked at physiological and psychological responses when people view imagery of nature—comparing natural to urban scenes, real plants to fake ones, and even pots containing flowers or bamboo to those without—and found physiologic responses to nature across the board. Again, these changes include improvements in heart rate and blood pressure, but also a positive effect on oxyhemoglobin concentrations in the prefrontal cortex, which is associated with a relaxed state.[40]

Nature and Exercise

There it is again: the prefrontal cortex, the hero of the story. I thought my brain was addicted to running, enthralled by the excitement and adventure of mountaineering, that it was still driven by primitive urges coming from the limbic system. But *nature* was the common thread between these sports. After living in Colorado, my relationship with the treadmill went from love to hate, and we broke up. Running on a treadmill was painfully boring, and I no longer bought into the popular misconception that running on a treadmill is easier than running outside. Once a "gym rat," I became an outdoor runner. I could not stare at the digital display or breathe the stuffy air in the gym anymore; I needed to feel the breeze on my face, listen to the crunch of leaves beneath my feet, and see the horizon in front of me. Even on the worst weather days, when rain cascaded down my clothes and into my shoes, when East Coast humidity wrapped around me like a wet blanket, I chose to run outside. Every time I exercised outside, I was strengthening my prefrontal cortex. If running was like weightlifting for my prefrontal cortex, bulking it up with each repetition, then nature was the protein shake, the added ingredient that made the workout stronger.

Access to green spaces makes people more likely to exercise outside—cycling, running, walking, hiking—and those activities are often done for a longer period than they would be in a gym.[41]

This provides a boost to the physiologic benefits that come with being in nature. Combining exercise with nature can enhance learning and memory and enrich the experience of physical activity. Nature provides an extra layer that makes exercise more interesting and engaging—changes in scenery, obstacles that don't exist on a treadmill, sensory integration with the sounds and smells of nature.

There is even some evidence to suggest that exercise feels easier when performed in a natural environment.[42] When allowed to self-select walking speed, people tend to walk faster outdoors than they do indoors. Paradoxically, they report lower perceived exertion. The same holds true in trained athletes—for example, ultramarathoners—who are able to exercise at higher intensities and for a longer duration when in nature.

While both indoor and outdoor exercise are beneficial for physical and mental health, studies show that outdoor athletes enjoy it more and report less anxiety afterward.[43] This is likely due to a combination of factors—our brains are churning out endogenous opioids and endocannabinoids, and we are engaging in a natural environment that distracts us from negative emotions and sensation of pain—that minimize the perception of effort. If we perceive exercise to be easier, and if we actually enjoy it, we're more likely to do it again and for longer.

Nature as Therapy

As I mentioned, one therapy used to treat eating disorders is biofeedback therapy. It can also be used to treat ADHD, PTSD, phobias, migraines, and chronic pain syndromes. In the face of stress or pain, the nervous system initiates a succession of involuntary responses in the body, such as increased heart rate, increased blood pressure, muscle tension, sweating, and temperature changes. Imagine something you fear—spiders, public speaking, a plane crash—and you can feel some of these changes in your body without measuring them.

Biofeedback is a method to gain conscious control over the involuntary processes that occur in response to stress. In a controlled environment, sensors are used to measure the body's reaction to stress while the patient practices things like mindful meditation, deep breathing, muscle relaxation, and guided imagery to decrease their physiologic stress response. Deep breathing, for instance, can lower your respiratory rate, which can lessen anxiety and produce a feeling of calm. But you don't have to be in a controlled environment to learn or practice biofeedback; you can practice deep breathing and meditation anywhere, including while walking through a forest, sitting on a beach, or wandering through a garden.

Based on what we know about nature's effects on mental and physical health, it is no surprise that nature has become a part of the healing process for many people. Nature-based health interventions (NBIs), sometimes called ecotherapy, are programs that engage people with nature to improve mental health and well-being. NBIs include horticultural therapy, which involves anything from digging in a garden to observing plants while sitting on a park bench, activities that lessen anxiety; wilderness therapy, which includes camping, learning survival skills, and trying adventurous activities that promote self-discovery; and forest bathing. In cities, NBIs can take the form of biking or walking paths, community gardens, and installation of plants in indoor settings. Even in hospitals, simply having indoor plants and setting hospital beds to face a window can make a difference in alleviating pain and speeding up recovery.[44]

In Colorado, my ecotherapy was hiking and running, no

therapist needed. My co-pay went to REI, where I bought my first pair of Merrell hiking boots. From there, my appreciation of nature grew in parallel with my mental well-being and physical endurance.

Some of my favorite moments from races and mountaineering expeditions have had nothing to do with exercise and everything to do with nature. Watching the sunrise at the top of Mount Rainier, sleeping next to the glacial runoff on Mount Baker, feeling the sunlight stream through the trees on the Batona Trail. Those were the most peaceful moments, the moments that told me I was where I belonged and made me feel calm and content, removed from the stress of everyday life. I felt connected to nature in a way that transcended my love of sports. Outside of endurance sports, I have found nature by backpacking and camping with Rich in the Grand Tetons, snowshoeing alone in Rocky Mountain National Park, and visiting the national parks of Alaska and Utah with my mom. There seems to be a dose-dependent relationship with nature; the more I get, the more I want. And others agree, including cognitive psychologist David Sawyer, who coined the term "3-day effect" while studying the effects of prolonged nature immersion on cognition. He found that backpackers immersed in nature for four days felt a "neural reboot" around the three-day mark.[45]

I know that not everyone can have these experiences; travel and mountaineering trips cost money, and even good running shoes are expensive. If I were not a doctor, I might not have been able to afford the things that saved my mental health, especially a cross-country move to the beautiful state of Colorado. People who live in poverty or with lower economic status already face greater health challenges compared to those with higher incomes, including limited access to healthcare and nutritious food. In urban areas, these challenges are compounded by inequitable distribution of and access to green spaces. Many people are confined to small apartments and crowded neighborhoods without the means or transportation to get outside the city. So the people who might benefit most from exposure to nature often experience the least of it. In fact, in looking at health outcomes, a review of ninety studies found that individuals with lower socioeconomic status benefit more from exposure to nature than those with higher socioeconomic status.[46]

I know what it's like to feel trapped in a city and to be trapped by mental illness. It's hard to imagine anything beyond the wilting potted trees and sickly pigeons that line the sidewalks. But nature experiences can still exist, even within the constraints of urban life. Nature-based interventions are everywhere—in city parks and gardens, in the art and photography displayed in museums, as a part of biophilic designs inside buildings and restaurants—if you look for them.

When I lived in Philly, a cheap pair of sneakers opened my eyes to my own potential as an athlete and gave me a chance to escape city life and breathe the unfiltered air. It wasn't always *fresh* air—sometimes it reeked of garbage and smog—but it was better than being stifled indoors. I went from running on city streets to running on trails to climbing glaciated mountains. My footwear evolved with my love of nature, from beat-up sneakers to trail-running shoes to hiking boots and eventually crampons. But my purpose in wearing them was always the same: I wanted to feel the earth beneath my feet, to be part of the natural world around me. I felt the earth all the way to the top of Mount Rainier, and I would feel it with every step of my longest race yet.

Chapter 19

THE PERFECT TEST

"What are your goals for this race? What do you want to accomplish?" my running coach, Genevieve, asked a few days before the MST Endurance Run, a race along the Mountains-to-Sea Trail across North Carolina. These were the same questions I asked myself every time I ran a race, but this time I was going into it wise to the things that motivated me. It wasn't beating a time goal or avoiding a DNF. And it definitely wasn't winning—I was slow, and at the age of thirty-eight, I would never be at the head of the pack. I was taking all the lessons I had learned about running and about myself—now a self-proclaimed endurance athlete, exercise junkie, nature enthusiast, and eating disorder survivor—to the starting line of my first 50-mile race.

I had met Genevieve after the Batona ultramarathon. Although it was only my second ultra, I felt strong and unstoppable after that race, not only as a runner but as someone who had overcome a serious mental health disorder. The risk of relapse was not a threat anymore. I could open the refrigerator without anxiety and choose a healthful snack without fear of bingeing. I could look in the mirror and see my body as powerful and healthy. I was liberated from the depression and anxiety that had been tethered to my eating disorder for so many years. Instead of looking back at the past, I was forging ahead as an athlete, making my own destiny.

As a runner, the path ahead could be whatever I wanted it to be. The path to becoming a doctor had been a long, straight line, and most of us ended up in the same place—practicing in offices and hospitals, collecting nice paychecks and luxury cars. But running was different. In a world of multiple choice, it was an open-ended question. The future was not as black and white as I once thought it was. I didn't need a coach to tell me to put my sneakers on; I needed someone to know my story to help unlock an even greater potential that existed within me.

Team RunRun offers remote coaching from athletes all across the country, and Genevieve was based in my favorite place: Colorado. She was a professional ultramarathoner who excelled at the 100-mile distance and even set a running "FKT" (fastest known time) on Mount Elbert, Colorado's highest peak. She was warm and down to earth, and I immediately clicked with her. On our first meeting, she asked, "What does running mean to you? Why do you love to run?" No one had ever asked me that before, and it was suddenly hard to put into words. There was a lump in my throat as I told her my story, how running brought me peace and empowered my recovery. I had never spoken those words freely to a complete stranger, but I felt like I could trust her. I was surprised that she seemed a bit choked up too; she was an empath, and I knew she would be a great coach for me.

We got to work, building speed intervals and hill workouts into my existing training regimen. I tracked my runs on a fitness app,

19 | THE PERFECT TEST

where she left motivating messages tagged to my workouts: "Strong work!" and "You are super fit!" Having a coach added a layer of accountability to my training and made me want to work a little harder each time. Metrics were important, but they weren't everything. Genevieve believed in quality over quantity, that accumulating miles and distance did not necessarily make you a better runner. But she wanted me to focus on running above all other forms of exercise. "The only way to become a better runner is to *run*," she said. Kickboxing and soccer would not help me at mile 40. We worked on nutrition plans and recovery and all the essentials that went into endurance racing. Then we tested out the training on my next ultra.

I signed up for the No Man's 50K Challenge in Virginia in March 2023. The race was created for female participants only, proof that more women were entering the sport of ultrarunning. In the days preceding the race, the East Coast was inundated with rain and wind. My mom and I drove to Virginia the night before the race, the storm pummeling my windshield, never relenting during the four-hour drive. It was following me, just as it had in Cool, California. I arrived already feeling weary.

The rain finally abated, leaving the trail muddy and slippery at 6 a.m. on race day, but despite bad trail conditions, I felt confident. Thanks to my coach, I was approaching the 50K distance better prepared than I had been in prior races. It was no longer a question of *if* I would finish; it was a matter of how fast and how strong.

The race comprised two hilly sixteen-mile loops through Prince William Forest Park, abutting Marine Corps Base Quantico. Within the first two miles of the race, soft beams of sunlight started to stream through the tops of beech trees, and I quickly shed my headlamp and gloves. The morning air was a crisp 40°F, the start of a beautiful, sunny winter day. I ran alongside Quantico

Creek, slowed by slippery downhills and large rocks along the water's edge, but my legs felt strong for the first loop. As I reached the halfway point, I saw my mom, one of the few spectators who stayed for the entire race. She cheered for me, offering extra energy gels and a bottle of Gatorade.

I was grateful to have her there. She was there for the most memorable moments in my life: birthday celebrations, soccer games, the day I moved away to college, graduations, the white coat ceremony before medical school, my first half-marathon, my wedding. She was there for the trivial moments too. She worried about me with every adventure and challenge I took on, but never warned me away from the attempt or doubted my ability. She believed in me. She gave me everything she had until I could stand on my own two feet as an adult, and that day she gave me Gatorade when my feet wanted to give out beneath me.

We had survived tough times together, and she was the parent who had stuck around no matter what. As I overcame my eating disorder, she defeated her alcohol addiction. She recovered, and then she rebuilt her life. She went back to school to earn a bachelor's degree, and then a master's degree in social work so she could counsel other people through trauma and conflict. Through years of individual therapy, she found balance in her own life again. She was back to being the selfless, loving mom I had always known, and she could even drink a glass of wine with me over dinner, the same way I could again eat a piece of cake without going off the deep end. Years after a cataclysmic divorce, she was stronger and more self-sufficient than ever.

Seeing her was a reminder of the mental toughness and perseverance I needed to finish the race. It was hard to start the second loop, to run back out on the trail away from the comforts of the start/finish line, but I forced myself to move. Each passing mile, marked by my Garmin watch, became a mental

19 | THE PERFECT TEST

countdown: *Only 15 miles to go; only 10 miles to go.* I willed my legs to keep moving. At mile 30, I crossed a small suspension bridge, and it bounced beneath me, sending shock waves up my achy legs.

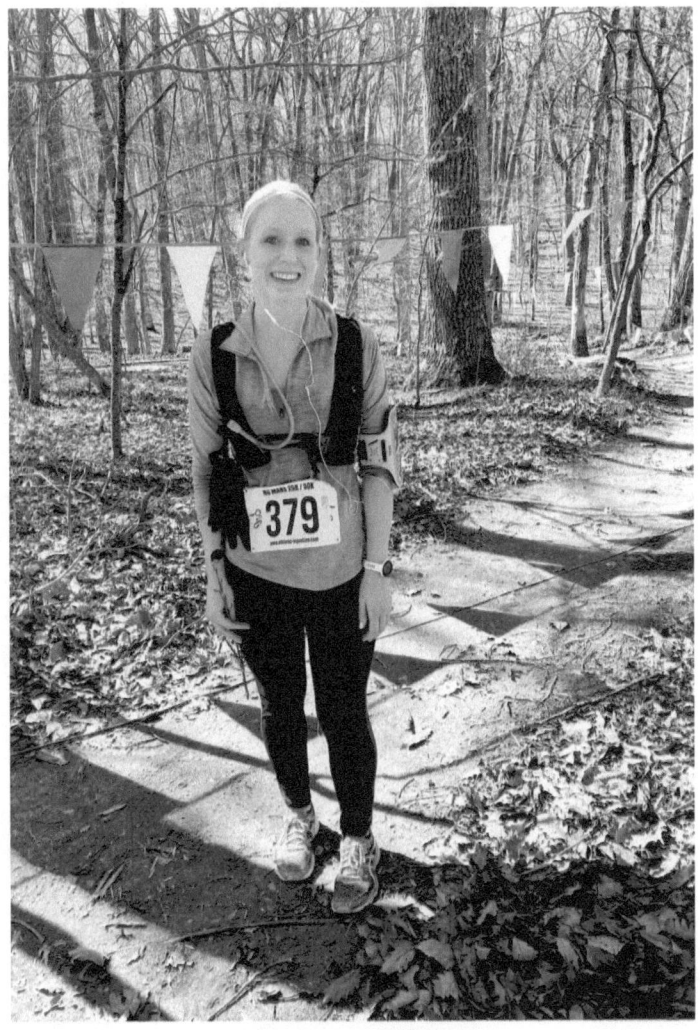

At the No-Man's 50K Challenge

I questioned what I was doing and why I was out there—the same questions I asked myself during every ultra before I reached the glorious finish line, remembered the answers, and forgot the pain. I wanted to cry out in anguish, to complain to anyone who would listen, but there was only silence from the canopy of trees and the boulders beside the trail. I was on my own; the forest had no compassion for my suffering. Then came another hill, and at last I could see the banner for the finish line waving in the breeze ahead. I gave one final push and finished in eighth place, my best performance yet.

A strong finish in another 50K. I was becoming consistent at a distance beyond the standard 26.2 miles. I was no longer plagued by imposter syndrome as a runner or as a doctor; I was capable, and I belonged at the start line of these races the same way I belonged in a white coat, reflex hammer in hand, examining patients with spinal cord injury and neuropathy. I wondered how much more I could give. When pushed to the limit, which would give up first—my body or my mind? Could I train my mind to make my body go even farther and faster up mountains and down trails?

Fifty miles. The words popped into my mind the same way the word "marathon" had, and then they stayed fixed there like boulders in a stream, rerouting the current, firmly rooted and refusing to budge. I had to try it. A 50-mile race would be the perfect way to test my physical and mental toughness.

The number was arbitrary—for someone else, it could have been one block, one mile, 5 kilometers, 26.2 miles, 100 kilometers, 100 miles. Extreme ultrarunners were out there running even longer distances. In the Marathon des Sables, runners traverse more than 250 kilometers in a multistage, multiday race across the Sahara Desert; in the ITI 1000, they follow the Iditarod trail for 1,000 miles across the blustery winter landscape of Alaska. Some runners travel across states, countries, and continents to set world records; others run the lengths of the longest trails in the country, like the Pacific Crest Trail or the Continental Divide Trail along the spine of the Rocky Mountains.

What mattered was that the distance was a personal challenge, and that it evoked enough awe and uncertainty that I wasn't sure if I could do it. For me, that distance was 50 miles. It was a highway commute to work, a train or bus ride to a city, a distance that seemed inconceivable on foot. An unattainable goal that I could inch closer to through hard work and discipline until it became attainable. I signed up for the MST Endurance Run. I had one year to train for it.

In the months leading up to the race, I challenged myself in new ways, signing up for races of varying distances that posed different obstacles. Some of them were cancelled before I hit the start line due to weather and other uncontrollable variables, so I got creative: I challenged the parts of my personality that had once defined me when I was anorexic and bulimic. If overachieving, award-winning Little Miss Perfect liked cheering fans and a medal at the end of a marathon, then I would run 26.2 miles by myself, against myself, in the woods. The day I did it, the weather was moody and irritable, but I didn't care. For all the times nature had accepted me as less than perfect, I accepted nature's imperfection in return.

It was early fall, and I was visiting my mom in Blairstown. Every time I visited Blairstown as an adult, I was surprised how little had changed. The same grocery store, the same pizza joints, the same gas stations and delis stayed open, but nothing new thrived. One of the town's greatest constants was the Paulinskill Valley Trail, a historical rail trail that stretched across Sussex and Warren Counties. On a sunny day, it was well traveled by runners, cyclists, and people walking their dogs, but on a cold, rainy day, I had it all to myself. I laced my sneakers and braced myself against the rain, which came down intermittently in slanted sheets.

I ran hard and splashed through puddles and mud. A mosaic of colorful leaves had already fallen, obscuring the ground and swishing beneath my feet. I passed landmarks from my childhood—a gnarled tree root where I had crashed my bike; the entrance to Footbridge Park, where the annual Fourth of July festival took place; a crossing where a black bear had stopped me in my tracks. As a kid, I had spent countless hours riding my bike on the trail with friends, sometimes stopping at the local airport cafe for a strawberry milkshake. As a teenager, I walked the trail at night with my sister and friends, spooked by the shadows and the glimmer of moonlight through the trees. When I was in medical school, training for my first half-marathon, I ran my first double-digit run there, at a time when running a half-marathon distance felt impossible. Twelve years later, I was racing along the same trail, flooded by rain and nostalgia. Mud caked my legs, and my socks squished with each step as I finished a marathon all by myself. Little Miss Perfect be damned.

Trail races are exciting, with new terrain and vistas around every turn. Some runners even seek out destination marathons and trail races as an excuse to do a road trip or get on an airplane. If my brain craved adventure and excitement the same way it once craved the thrill and impulsivity of binge eating, then I would choose to bore myself to tears, to prove that I could run

19 | THE PERFECT TEST

without those things motivating me. So for my next ultra, instead of a point-to-point race through a forested landscape, I ran in circles. It was a timed race, and the goal was to run as many 2.5-mile loops as possible in eight hours. To get to the race site, I had to drive through two hours of traffic on monotonous highways to a place that was as mundane as New Jersey: Pennsylvania. On the day of the race, in the middle of December, it was overcast and cold, making the repetitive loop of crushed gravel and dirt look even less beautiful. I was bored to death before it began.

My thoughts and the songs on my Apple Music playlist were the only things that changed as I ran counterclockwise loop after counterclockwise loop. Fatigue, stiffness, and rising lactic acid in my muscles were the only proof that I was going anywhere as I crossed the start/finish line over and over. But I did it. I ran 38 miles that day, one mile for each year I had been alive. More importantly, I embraced boredom, the enemy of the thrill seeker and adrenaline junkie in me.

I enjoyed these runs that challenged what I thought I knew about myself. They were etched into my memory as Type II fun, just as climbing Mount Rainier was. They were the stepping-stones to a bigger challenge, the savory appetizers before the entrée. And, in the end, they left me hungry for the main event.

Chapter 20

FIFTY MILES

The forecast held rain, and not just a little rain—a deluge. In the hospital, some doctors attract constant emergencies, sleepless call nights, crashing patients, and code blues; we call them "black clouds." I never earned that nickname at work, but I was definitely the black cloud of running. I do not exaggerate when I say that rain followed me wherever I ran. The day of the MST Endurance Run—perfectly sandwiched between two sunny, dry, early spring days—was saturated.

The Mountains-to-Sea Trail, stretching 1,175 miles across North Carolina from the Great Smoky Mountains to the Outer Banks, passes through three national forests and three national parks as the state's longest marked trail. My race, the MST 50-mile trail race, spanned one small length of it. But it was farther than I had ever run before. Even if my brain believed I could run that far, and my body agreed, fully committed to giving 100 percent effort to the task, would the weather, an injury, or some other unpredictable complication stop me anyway?

When we gathered at the start line just before 6 a.m., the rain had already begun, and I knew I was in for a long and painful day. But I was ready: I had run my first half-marathon over a decade earlier, I had run marathons and ultramarathons in the pouring rain, and I was a stronger and faster endurance runner than I had ever been in my twenties.

I took off in the darkness, my headlamp guiding the way from the paved road into the wet, primordial forest. It was a precarious game of "follow the leader," and when the first group of men made a wrong turn, I found myself leading them through the woods, around twists and turns on a trail I could barely see beneath my feet. For a few minutes, I felt the glory of being in first place, even if it was short-lived.

In the eerie gray light of the rainy morning, the white circular trail markers on the trees popped up like ghosts in a haunted forest every few hundred feet—the only guides in an otherwise directionless, disorienting maze. Unlike the No Man's 50K, there was no sun streaming through the trees, no beacon to light the way. The ground was slippery and uneven. I stepped carefully at first, trying to dodge puddles and exposed tree roots, but by mile 3, as my sneakers skied down a mud slick into an ankle-deep puddle, I knew it was futile. I was going to be drenched and muddy for the rest of the day, and I had to lean into it. The same puddles that slowed me down would slow everyone down; no one was immune. From then on, instead of skipping around the puddles or going off trail, I ran straight through them and let the mud splash up the sides of my legs.

I had two simple goals: Don't quit, and stay positive.

Positive thinking and the light of my headlamp carried me through the first few hours. By the time I reached the aid station at mile 17, my shorts were glued to my thighs, my sneakers were full of mud, and my earbuds were drenched. Pop music faded in and out, warped by the rain, and I wondered if my smart phone would drown before the race was over. But somehow, despite my pace being slowed to twelve-minute miles by the slippery mud, I led the women's group. I couldn't believe it. I had never come close to being in the lead at any race. That morale boost helped keep my thoughts positive as the rain continued to fall. Without wasting any time, I grabbed my favorite aid station food—a peanut butter and jelly sandwich—and got back on the trail.

The course was two out-and-back segments, one 16 miles total and the other 34 miles total. We started on the larger segment, and I was now on the 17-mile stretch back toward the start line where I would cross to the smaller segment for the final third of the race. Now that hours of rain had accumulated on the trail and turned it into a rivulet, every obstacle I had faced on the way out was ten times worse heading back. Every uphill became a strenuous hike, as my legs splayed out in the slick mud with each step, and I desperately grasped onto tree branches to maintain balance. The muddy earth sucked at my sneakers hungrily, trying to devour one shoelace at a time like loose spaghetti strands. At times it felt like I was surfing or skiing, riding the waves of mud, rather than running. A pulled muscle or sprained ankle felt inevitable. But I kept going, and I kept the lead until the marathon distance had passed. *I won!* I thought, celebrating a small victory in my head. There was no award for first place at 26.2 miles though; we were just past the halfway point.

"What can I get you?" she asked. "Do you need more water? We have pancakes, donuts, sports massages, whatever you need." I was back at the start line, mile 34, and was ushered into the warm community building by a support crew member. I eyed her enviously, dressed in dry clothes with her long blonde hair neat and straight down her back. My ponytail was now thick with knots, as untamed as a wild horse's, clinging to the nape of my neck.

I looked around the room. Some runners were getting massages; others had teams of family members and spouses changing their socks and refilling their hydration packs like pit crews at a NASCAR race. Support staff walked around offering up electrolyte drinks like they were glasses of champagne at a gala. It was the most glorious aid station I had ever seen. How luxurious would it be to sit down with a plate of pancakes and warm up my feet, to give in to temptation and just stop running completely?

Genevieve had warned me that coming back to the start line two-thirds of the way through the race would be dangerous. It felt like the race was over, but it wasn't. I had to ignore the enticement of being indoors again and go back out into the rain. I was by myself—my support crew was far away in New Jersey—and I had to push on solo. Without sitting down, I took a few minutes to rest and put on a fresh pair of socks, fully knowing they would be soaked through again as soon as I hit the trail, then jogged across the start line once more to commence the last 16 miles.

More mud, more rain, more pain. My legs strained as I walked uphill to the next aid station. My fresh socks were now soggy and coated in mud. "What mile marker is this?" I asked the aid station volunteer, grabbing a handful of orange slices and chips. "Thirty-nine," he replied, and my face fell. My Garmin watch, dead after nine hours of running, had lied. I thought I was at mile 41, and the disappointment felt as heavy as my wet clothes. On any normal day, on fresh legs, a two-mile difference wouldn't matter, but today it mattered a lot. I felt my resolve crumbling, and as I walked away from the aid station, I choked back tears. The wild swings of emotion, the highs and lows that came with ultrarunning, were finally catching up with me.

I called home, needing to hear Rich's voice. "You can do this," he urged. "You've trained so hard, and this means so much to you. Don't give up." His calming voice soothed me. "Stay on the phone with me another minute," I pleaded. There was a short river crossing up ahead, where the rain had transformed a stream into a swift current. My quads whined as I descended the sandy embankment and waded into the water, feeling its pull against my wobbly legs. Fearful of being knocked over and with nothing to hold on to, I fought against the current. "I'm not quitting," I said, my voice thick with the threat of tears. "I'm going to get this done." Moments later, I was out of the water and climbing up the opposite bank to get back on the trail.

Although I was by myself on the trail for miles at a time, I never felt alone. There were incoming text messages with words of encouragement from my family and friends. I spoke to my mom and sister, letting their enthusiasm drown out the din of the rain for a few minutes. So many people supported and loved me; they had always been there for me. Why hadn't sixteen-year-old me turned to them when she needed help?

I also crossed paths with other runners I had met that morning. There was a woman about my age, who had come from Texas to run her ninth 100-mile race. We talked before the race and didn't see each other again until mile 42, as I was turning back toward the finish line. Through the night, she would continue to run another 50 miles while I slept soundly back in my hotel room. We didn't know each other by name, but we knew each other's origin stories. "You've got this, New Jersey!" she said. "I'm counting on you to get second place." The woman who had taken the lead at mile 29 was far ahead of me by now.

With seven miles to go, I felt like I could no longer run. I slowed to a walk and let my shoes sink deeper into the mud with each step. I had never felt so much pain in my legs, not even at the summit of Mount Rainier. I was convinced I needed to stop moving. But was it my body giving up, or my mind?

Sports psychologists call the idea that we mentally limit ourselves before we hit our physical limit the "central governor theory." Our bodies are capable of pushing harder than we ever think possible. The brain tells us to stop as a protective mechanism, a way to hit the brakes on physical exertion before we get sick or injured. But after training my body to run far, nourishing and hydrating it, and taking care of it for years after my recovery, did I need to hit the brakes? I could push through pain and quiet the negative thoughts telling me to stop. Pushing through is a way to overcome obstacles and build resilience, to strengthen the prefrontal cortex. It turns a solid red stop light into a flashing yellow, and eventually, into green.

I wasn't sick or injured; I was just *tired*. Tired of trudging through the mud and being soaked by the rain. But I could still go on, one tired step at a time.

I thought of a conversation I'd had with my coach days before. Genevieve told me I would retreat into a "pain cave" during the race, and I knew exactly what she meant. The pain cave is a dark, isolating, deeply personal mental space, where pain overshadows any other emotion or sensation. Many ultrarunners, as well as people with depression, PTSD, and addiction, have been there. But I did not have to stay there; I could keep moving toward the light. "I know pain is transient," I told her. "And nothing can ever be as painful as the shame and sadness I felt with my eating disorder."

I thought back to that terrible night in residency—the shameful, wild night of excessive partying, drinking, and bingeing that left me crying on the bathroom floor with dried mascara on my cheeks and powdered sugar on my lips. The night that hurtled me toward recovery, desperate to escape the fate that awaited me if I stayed bulimic for the rest of my life. That was the deepest pain cave I had ever entered, and somehow I had crawled out of it and started to walk again and then run. If I could get through that, I could get through anything.

Even if I didn't run another step, I would walk and hike my way to the finish line. I walked for a while, slowly moving forward but never stopping, listening to my sneakers squish in the mud, until there was a renewed desire to run. First, I jogged a few steps, then the length of a switchback, then an entire song on my playlist. I refused to give up, mentally or physically. The miles crept by slowly, but each step brought me closer to the finish line. Around 6 p.m., twelve hours after I had begun my journey, I saw the road through the trees. Flat, even pavement had never looked so beautiful.

The trail-road conjunction marked the final mile of the race, the home stretch toward the finish line. I imagined the final mile of the Philadelphia Marathon, where the cheers of the crowds grew louder, and I pushed a little harder. I imagined running toward the finish line of every trail race I had ever run, taking the last satisfying steps toward the summit of Mount Rainier, sprinting toward the goal on a breakaway during a varsity soccer game. Those were the moments when I gave 110 percent of myself, when I dug deep to find that last bit of energy I didn't know existed.

At mile 49, I really *ran*. I ran faster than I had at the start of the race. I opened up my stride and pushed hard for the last mile, each footstrike on the pavement reverberating through my body, each breath ragged and labored. But oddly, it felt good. I was accomplishing something I had never thought possible, and that stoked a fire within me that warmed my waterlogged limbs and renewed my strength.

I crossed the finish line in twelve hours and twenty minutes, taking third place for the women and sixteenth overall. But in my mind, I won.

In my story, I had outrun perfection and broken the tape.

AFTERWORD

I am on a mountain again, but this time I am a thousand miles southeast of Mount Rainier, and nowhere near the summit. Mount Whitney stands tall at 14,505 feet, the crown jewel of the Sierra Nevada mountain range. It is a beautiful and statuesque mountain, but it can be moody.

When we started the climb yesterday, the blue sky was dotted with fluffy white cotton-ball clouds and the air was still. Even in fifty-degree weather, I was sweating through my base layer after the first mile of uphill climbing, and my 50-pound pack felt as if it were glued to my skin. I was carrying the extra weight of a group tent, snowshoes, heavier mountaineering boots, and a hefty container of gnocchi and marinara sauce for our group's dinner, but I refused to look burdened by it. If the men could carry the weight, so could I.

Seven hours of snowshoeing later, we arrived at a flat area of snow and then painstakingly assembled base camp. Wind whipped through camp as we dug makeshift tent stakes—snowshoes, ice axes, tree branches, rocks, anything that could be repurposed—into the frozen ground. We were a group of six, led by two guides from Sierra Mountaineering International. "See that?" Our guide Ben pointed upward. "That's a lenticular cloud." I captured it on camera, high above the heads of my fellow climbers. Little did we know that the whimsical saucer-shaped cloud was a sign of the impending snowstorm.

The night grew cold as 40 mph winds battered the sides of the tents. Zero-degree sleeping bags, down jackets, and all-weather tents, which we thought were impenetrable, were no match for the cold. We had a sleepless night listening to the cacophony of the storm.

By breakfast, the weather was calm again, and we decided to move up the mountain toward camp two. That decision seemed to anger the mountain. Within a few hours, the snow fell heavily, the wind gusted, and the summit of Mount Whitney disappeared behind a wall of spindrift. The avalanche risk was growing by the minute, and the mountain was pushing back against our progress up its snowy slopes.

The guides turned us back at 11,500 feet, only two days into the trip and thousands of feet shy of the summit.

We are now making our way back down to the base of the mountain, and the descent is even more arduous. My snowshoes splay out in an effort to keep my balance on the steep terrain, and I can feel my quads burning from the strain of constant braking. It is the type of burning pain that will last for days, probably until I am back home in New Jersey. I know this pain well. I feel like I'm skiing when I'd rather not be, dangerously close to a ravine that parallels the path through the trees. There is no trail to follow, only the footsteps of the person in front of me. I look down across the snowy slope and catch my breath, steadying the heavy pack on my shoulders.

Although we didn't make the summit, I am not disappointed. For someone running from perfection, it is a fitting ending to the

AFTERWORD

trip. Not every climb ends in a summit, and I have other things to be grateful for: I'm immersed in nature at its wildest. I'm doing something I love, throwing all my physical and mental effort into an endurance sport. I'm sweaty and dirty, my unbrushed hair is sticking out from beneath my winter hat, and my nose is running, but I feel beautiful and untamed, as majestic as the mountain herself. Every step I have taken has been effortful. I am tired, but the physical strain of climbing comes nowhere close to the emotional pain and shame I battled with my eating disorder.

For fourteen years of my life, I was *sick*. Not the obvious kind of sick that comes with intravenous infusions, blood draws, prolonged hospital stays, bouquets of flowers, and get-well cards. My sickness was literally in my mind. I was plagued by an invisible monster, the eating disorder that followed me wherever I went. In residency, bulimia magnified the stress that came with eighty-hour workweeks and sleepless nights, and recovery felt damn near impossible.

Eventually, I became my own doctor and psychoanalyst; I found my willpower and the ability to make a choice. I chose to get better, just as I chose to make it to med school commencement and eventually to the finish line of a 50-mile race and the summit of Mount Rainier. Nature and exercise facilitated my recovery. Running empowered me to view my body as capable and beautiful, something I never thought possible when I was anorexic, when running a mile on the treadmill at the Lehigh gym felt like summiting Mount Everest. Mountaineering gave me peace and brought me closer to nature. As a neurologist who has studied her own brain, I have finally figured out what draws me to these sports: Endurance sports are food for my mind and soul. They make me *happy*, and that is reason enough to pursue them. Now, when I stand at a patient's bedside, I don't have to pretend: I exemplify health.

I spent too many years of my life trying to be perfect—the perfect student, the perfect daughter, the girl with the perfect body. I got lost in a world of rigid thinking and rules, and impossible standards I set for myself. I worried too much about the number on the scale; now I care more about the weight of my pack. As I transitioned from running on roads to running on dirt trails and climbing mountains, I realized why I love trails and mountains so much: They are imperfect, and unapologetic about it. Trails are not smooth and linear; they are unpredictable and challenging. On the surface they might be crumbling and eroded, but underneath is a strong, immovable foundation. Sometimes a tree root catches your toe or a steep, muddy hill forces you to crawl. You might twist an ankle and take a fall, and the hard dirt and rocks below refuse to coddle you. They leave you bleeding and exposed, but a little tougher as you take the next step forward. Letting go of perfection allowed me to be free, and to take twists and turns in stride. It allowed me to see the beauty in the imperfections of my own body.

I continue down the snowy slope, one slippery step at a time, snowflakes bouncing off my goggles and melting into the sweat that runs down my temples. My muscles are ready for a break, but my mind convinces them to persist. Once again, I am amazed by my body's ability to endure, and my mind's ability to command it to do incredible things.

I will appreciate every moment I have in this body, regardless of what it looks like. I no longer need a mirror to see it. I find my reflection in alpine lakes and glaciers, in the granite fortresses I climb, in the wild landscapes I run through. I will continue to run for myself, away from perfection, always toward the sunlight, and let the shadows fall behind me.

AFTERWORD

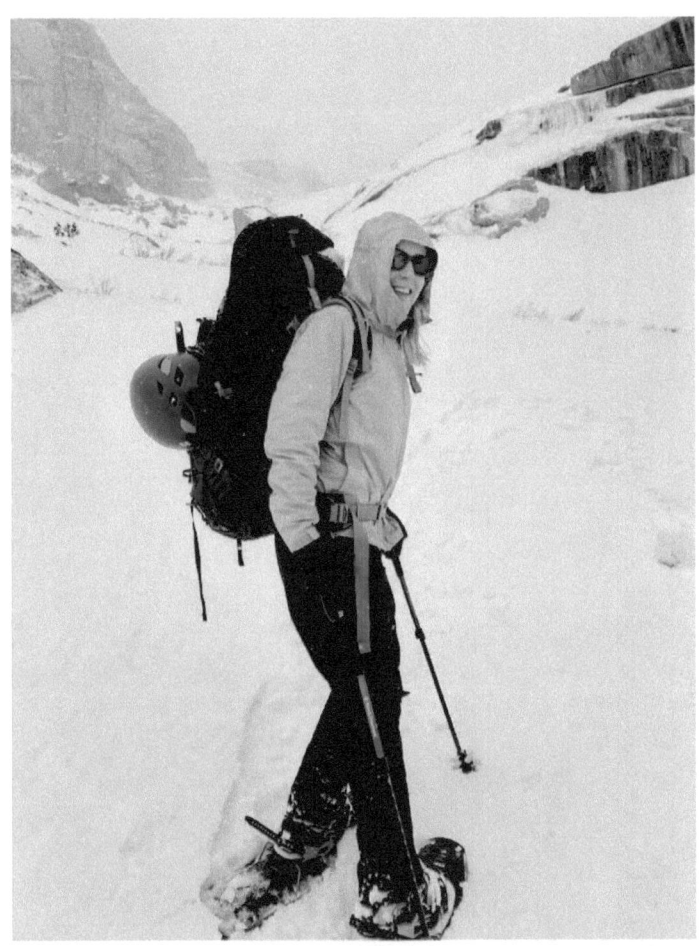

Mount Whitney

ACKNOWLEDGMENTS

First and foremost, thank you to my mom for being a role model of perseverance and resilience. You've always encouraged me to follow my dreams, no matter how crazy they may seem in the moment. With your love and support, I've achieved more than I ever thought possible. I hope I always make you proud.

To my husband, Rich, my soulmate, my twin flame—you were the first person to know my truth. Without you, I never would have shared my story. Thank you for loving me despite my flaws, even though you pretend not to see them. I'll always be your "Little Miss Perfect." Thank you for supporting every aspiration—from running ultramarathons to mountaineering to pursuing another college degree—because you know how much I love a project.

Thank you to my sister, Kerin, and my brother, Stephen, for your love, protection, and friendship. What our family lacks in size, it makes up for in fierce loyalty.

To my best friend, Jen—you have been by my side throughout the writing of this book, an unofficial editor, and you inspired the title. I can't thank you enough.

I am lucky to have met many positive female role models who played a part in my recovery—Erin, Danielle, and others not mentioned by name in this book. Thank you for showing me how to be healthy, athletic, and strong. You did this effortlessly and unintentionally and led by example.

To my coach, Genevieve—thank you for making me a stronger athlete. Your gentle guidance and motivating words have led me to personal bests and distances I never thought I'd run.

To the team at Clear Sight Books, especially my editor, Karin Wiberg—thank you for believing in me as a new author. It was a childhood dream to be a writer, and that dream got buried beneath a pile of ambitions and degrees; when I felt brave enough to share my story, you helped me bring it back to the surface. Thank you for guiding me on this incredible, transformative journey.

Lastly, I am grateful for my dog Chief, who passed away before this book was published. He was my faithful writing companion, napping next to my laptop and peeking over the screen when he decided it was time for a walk. He will be forever missed.

NOTES

[1] "General Eating Disorder Statistics," National Eating Disorders Association.

[2] Jon Arcelus et al., "Mortality Rates in Patients with Anorexia Nervosa and Other Eating Disorders. A Meta-Analysis of 36 Studies," *Archives of General Psychiatry* 68, no. 7, 2011.

[3] J. M. Harlow and Edgar Miller, "Recovery from the Passage of an Iron Bar Through the Head," *History of Psychiatry* 4, no. 14, 1993.

[4] Laramie Duncan et al., "Significant Locus and Metabolic Genetic Correlations Revealed in Genome-Wide Association Study of Anorexia Nervosa," *American Journal of Psychiatry* 174, no. 9, 2017.

[5] Laura M. Thornton et al., "The Heritability of Eating Disorders: Methods and Current Findings," *Current Topics in Behavioral Neurosciences* 6, 2011.

[6] Duncan, "Significant Locus."

[7] Dianne Neumark-Sztainer et al., "Family Weight Talk and Dieting: How Much Do They Matter for Body Dissatisfaction and Disordered Eating Behaviors In Adolescent Girls?" *Journal of Adolescent Health* 47, no. 3, 2010.

[8] Laurie Dufresne et al., "Personality Traits in Adolescents with Eating Disorder: A Meta-Analytic Review," *International Journal of Eating Disorders* 53, no. 2, 2020.

[9] Lucy M. Dahill et al., "Associations Between Parents' Body Weight/Shape Comments and Disordered Eating Amongst Adolescents over Time—A Longitudinal Study," *Nutrients* 15, no. 6, 2023.

[10] Norman J. Temple, "The Origins of the Obesity Epidemic in the USA-Lessons for Today," *Nutrients* 14, no. 20, 2022.

[11] Shirley B. Wang et al., "Fifteen-Year Prevalence, Trajectories, and Predictors of Body Dissatisfaction from Adolescence to Middle Adulthood," *Clinical Psychological Science* 7, no. 6, 2019.

[12] *Diagnostic and Statistical Manual of Mental Disorders*, Fifth Edition, Text Revision (DSM-5-TR), American Psychiatric Association, 2022.

[13] DSM-5-TR.

[14] Leah M. Kalm and Richard D. Semba, "They Starved So That Others Be Better Fed: Remembering Ancel Keys and the Minnesota Experiment," *The Journal of Nutrition* 135, no. 6, 2005.

[15] Kesha Baptiste-Roberts and Mian Hossain, "Socioeconomic Disparities and Self-Reported Substance Abuse-Related Problems," *Addiction & Health* 10, no. 2, 2018.

[16] Howard Steiger, "Eating Disorders and the Serotonin Connection: State, Trait and Developmental Effects," *Journal of Psychiatry & Neuroscience* 29, no. 1, 2004.

[17] Walter H. Kaye et al., "Comorbidity of Anxiety Disorders with Anorexia and Bulimia Nervosa," *The American Journal of Psychiatry* 161, no. 12, 2004.

[18] Tamara Berends et al., "Relapse in Anorexia Nervosa: A Systematic Review and Meta-Analysis," *Current Opinion in Psychiatry* 31, no. 6, 2018.

[19] Stein Frostad et al., "BMI at Discharge from Treatment Predicts Relapse in Anorexia Nervosa: A Systematic Scoping Review," *Journal of Personalized Medicine* 12, no. 5, 2022.

[20] Vivienne M. Hazzard et al., "Food Insecurity and Eating Disorders: A Review of Emerging Evidence," *Current Psychiatry Reports* 22, no. 12, 2020.

[21] Jenny H. Conviser et al., "Essentials for Best Practice: Treatment Approaches for Athletes with Eating Disorders," *Journal of Clinical Sport Psychology* 12, no. 4, 2018.

[22] Ryley Mancine et al., "Disordered Eating and Eating Disorders in Adolescent Athletes," *Spartan Medical Research Journal* 4, no. 2, 2020.

[23] Christina M. Sanzari et al., "The Impact of Social Media Use on Body Image and Disordered Eating Behaviors: Content Matters More than Duration of Exposure," *Eating Behaviors* 49, 2023.

[24] Hamdi Yılmaz et al., "Association of Orthorexic Tendencies with Obsessive-Compulsive Symptoms, Eating Attitudes and Exercise," *Neuropsychiatric Disease and Treatment* 16, 2020.

[25] Jonathan R. Scarff, "Orthorexia Nervosa: An Obsession with Healthy Eating," *Federal Practitioner* 34, no. 6, 2017.

[26] National Eating Disorders Association, Eating Disorders Screening Tool.

[27] Rachael E. Flatt et al., "Comparing Eating Disorder Characteristics and Treatment in Self-Identified Competitive Athletes and Non-Athletes from the National Eating Disorders Association Online Screening Tool," *International Journal of Eating Disorders* 54, no. 3, 2020.

²⁸ Mancine, "Disordered Eating."
²⁹ Margaret Catherine Macpherson et al., "Investigating Coaches' Recognition of Symptoms of Eating Disorders in Track Athletes," *BMJ Open Sport & Exercise Medicine* 8, no. 3, 2022.
³⁰ Gregory S. Roebuck et al., "The Psychology of Ultramarathon Runners: A Systematic Review," *Psychology of Sport and Exercise* 37, 2018.
³¹ Josine E. Verhoeven et al., "Antidepressants or Running Therapy: Comparing Effects on Mental and Physical Health in Patients with Depression and Anxiety Disorders," *Journal of Affective Disorders* 329, 2023.
³² Matthew Pearce et al., "Association Between Physical Activity and Risk of Depression: A Systematic Review and Meta-Analysis," *JAMA Psychiatry* 79, no. 6, 2022.
³³ J. Peen et al., "The Current Status of Urban-Rural Differences in Psychiatric Disorders," *Acta Psychiatrica Scandinavica* 121, 2010.
³⁴ Gus Stahl, "Health Impact: The Pros and Cons of Living in a City," *Global Citizen*, 2015.
³⁵ Jason Blevins, "Nearly Half of Americans Didn't Go Outside to Recreate in 2018. That Has the Outdoor Industry Worried," *The Colorado Sun*, January 29, 2020.
³⁶ Michelle C. Kondo et al., "Does Spending Time Outdoors Reduce Stress? A Review of Real-Time Stress Response to Outdoor Environments," *Health & Place* 51, 2018.
³⁷ Hyunju Jo et al., "Physiological Benefits of Viewing Nature: A Systematic Review of Indoor Experiments," *International Journal of Environmental Research and Public Health* 16, no. 23, 2019.
³⁸ Jo, "Physiological Benefits."
³⁹ Frances E. Kuo and Andrea Faber Taylor, "A Potential Natural Treatment for Attention-Deficit/Hyperactivity Disorder: Evidence from a National Study," *American Journal of Public Health* 94, no. 9, 2004.
⁴⁰ Jo, "Physiological Benefits."
⁴¹ Valerie F. Gladwell et al., "The Great Outdoors: How a Green Exercise Environment Can Benefit All," *Extreme Physiology & Medicine* 2, no. 1, 2013.
⁴² Gladwell, "The Great Outdoors."
⁴³ Gladwell, "The Great Outdoors."
⁴⁴ Danielle F. Shanahan et al., "Nature-Based Interventions for Improving Health and Wellbeing: The Purpose, the People and the Outcomes," *Sports* 7, no. 6, 2019.

[45] Matt Berry, "The 3-Day Effect: How Reconnecting with Nature Can Aid Your Recovery," American Addiction Centers, updated May 2, 2023.

[46] Marcia P. Jimenez et al., "Associations Between Nature Exposure and Health: A Review of the Evidence," *International Journal of Environmental Research and Public Health* 18, no. 9, 2021.

RESOURCES

Crisis Support

If you or someone you know is dealing with an eating disorder or other crisis, please reach out for support.

988 Suicide & Crisis Lifeline
https://988lifeline.org/
Call or text 988, or chat online, available 24/7

National Alliance for Eating Disorders
https://www.allianceforeatingdisorders.com/
Helpline: 1-866-662-1235, 9 a.m. to 7 p.m. Eastern, Monday through Friday

National Association of Anorexia Nervosa and Associated Disorders (ANAD)
https://anad.org/
Helpline: 1-888-375-7767, 9 a.m. to 9 p.m. Central, Monday through Friday

National Eating Disorders Association
https://www.nationaleatingdisorders.org/

Recommended Reading

Books on eating disorders:

An Apple a Day: A Memoir of Love and Recovery from Anorexia, Emma Woolf, Soft Skull, 2013.
Brain over Binge: Why I Was Bulimic, Why Conventional Therapy Didn't Work, and How I Recovered for Good, 2nd ed., Kathryn Hansen, Camellia Publishing, 2022.
Empty: A Memoir, Susan Burton, Random House, 2020.
Good Girls: A Story and Study of Anorexia, Hadley Freeman, Simon & Schuster, 2023.

Books on women in athletics:

Choose Strong: The Choice That Changes Everything, Sally McRae, Self-published, 2023.
Finding Elevation: Fear and Courage on the World's Most Dangerous Mountain, Lisa Thompson, Girl Friday Books, 2023.
The Girl Who Climbed Everest: Lessons Learned Facing Up to the World's Toughest Mountains, Bonita Norris, Hodder & Stoughton, 2018.
Good for a Girl: A Woman Running in a Man's World, Lauren Fleshman, Penguin, 2023.
Out and Back: A Runner's Story of Survival Against All Odds, Hillary Allen, Blue Star, 2021.

About the Author

CAITLIN MASSONE, MD, is a neurologist who specializes in treating patients with cerebrovascular disease. When she's not working, she's running, hiking, camping, skiing—anything outdoors—and is currently training to climb Denali. She lives in New Jersey with her husband, Rich, four stepchildren, and their rescue dog, Daisy.

www.ingramcontent.com/pod-product-compliance
Lightning Source LLC
Chambersburg PA
CBHW030442090526
44586CB00044B/518